WITHOUT
HELMETS
OR SHOULDER
PADS

WITHOUT HELMETS OR SHOULDER PADS

The American Way of Death in Football Conditioning

IRVIN MUCHNICK

Published by ECW Press
665 Gerrard Street East
Toronto, Ontario, Canada M4M 1Y2
416-694-3348 / info@ecwpress.com

Editor for the Press: Michael Holmes
Copy editor: Peter Norman
Cover design: David Drummond

LIBRARY AND ARCHIVES CANADA CATALOGUING
IN PUBLICATION

Title: Without helmets or shoulder pads : the American way of
death in football conditioning / Irvin Muchnick.

Names: Muchnick, Irvin, author.

Identifiers: Canadiana (print) 20230460518 | Canadiana (ebook)
20230460542

ISBN 978-1-77041-750-2 (softcover)
ISBN 978-1-77852-227-7 (ePub)
ISBN 978-1-77852-228-4 (PDF)
ISBN 978-1-77852-229-1 (Kindle)

Subjects: LCSH: Football injuries. | LCSH: Football injuries—
Patients. | LCSH: Football—Moral and ethical aspects.

Classification: LCC RC1220.F6 M83 2023 | DDC 617.1/0276332—
dc23

PRINTED AND BOUND IN CANADA

PRINTING: FRIESENS   5   4   3   2   1

Contents

Introduction

America's conversation over the fraught future of football, ongoing for a decade or more but also muted, has settled into an unacceptably low roar. Today it's nothing more than episodic background static. At this point, those of us who believe football, for all its popularity, is a blood sport wreaking unsustainable damage on national health — a historical blot analogous to the *panem et circenses* of the Roman Colosseum in the end game of another empire — have an obligation to do more than simply shout "CONCUSSION, CONCUSSION, CONCUSSION!" in a crowded theater.

The first step of a reset in examining football is to grasp how an existential critique of the nation's No. 1 sport stalled into tepid and purely cosmetic reforms, without changing the structure of the industry or the distribution of its participation and public subsidies. While acknowledging that football is entertaining, that it is resistant to being eradicated — and, indeed, cannot be eradicated simply because a minority are uncomfortable with it — we still need to be reevaluating the vectors that are truly controllable. Those include who plays and when and where.

Instead, we tinker with the sport's rules. Many such changes, like keeping the clock running in more situations and moving up the line for kickoffs, give away the game. By artificially reducing the number of real contested plays, these are tweaks that basically validate the argument against the sport's current universality. Is the end goal here really to make sure every individual contest now consists of a little less of a fundamentally hazardous thing? By analogy, high school boxing teams died out decades ago. Would it be OK for high schools still to have these teams so long as the length of each round were reduced?

The clock cheat and the reduction of the number of expected kickoff returns betray the larger reality that as dramatic as concussions are, an obsession with them has left other aspects of football harm on the table. In a bizarre way, the obsession actually helps let the sport off the hook. Thus was born this volume, thrusting under readers' noses an under-reported malodorous subset of football's variegated damage — and one deliberately chosen for its feature of having no component of contact trauma. By so *drilling down*, we can *arch up*, to the base story here of football's social power, its seemingly unchecked purchase on the American male soul.

Is the term "pandemic" appropriate for the scale of such deaths? Let's put it this way: football meets the rhetorical, if not the scientific, criteria. Our football pandemic is a socially induced one. It stems from a rite of passage pushed on boyly boys yearning to be manly men. As with rape and other phenomena that are hard to quantify with precision, largely because preexisting biases don't support such efforts, we can say that far more American males are killed or seriously harmed in football than the system is ever in the mood to measure. Reliably, we can float the number north of 700 teenagers who have died in high school football since some half-hearted tracking began in the 1930s. In college football, there have been up to three dozen deaths from attacks associated with the low-balled sickle cell genetic trait alone; these are set against the sobering backdrop that student-athletes are as much as four and a half times as likely to die non-traumatically, during conditioning, than they are from blocking and tackling during the games themselves.

A simultaneous American male problem here gets framed in more broadly pitched social commentary. By many measures, boys today are falling behind in school, and men in work life follow in their lagging footsteps. Growing up (or not), they drive metrics of "deaths of despair" and others of dysfunctions in relationships and child-rearing.

Yet, without a doubt, the spectacle of football endures and thrives; it's TV- and device-friendly, and diabolically conducive to the coast-to-coast expansion of above-board gambling, which our society used to confine to enclaves such as Las Vegas and Atlantic City. The American libertarian current runs deep and the human tropism for lookaway passes is powerful. Episodic evidence of late life mental deficits for famous football veterans is frighteningly real for the people who suffer them and for the loved ones who have to deal with them, but it also hands to apologists and fence-sitters the advantage of remaining ill-defined and abstract.

Those familiar with the traumatic brain injury (TBI) debate have long understood that the crowning argument about concussions should be that none of this was ever, in the first place, about concussions per se. The process leading to chronic traumatic encephalopathy (CTE), a condition by which deposits of tau protein cause the brain to lose impulse control and other basic functional regulations, results from an *accumulation* of blows — often dozens, scores, or hundreds of them across time, whether or not any of them met the clinical criteria or eye candy of concussions. Moreover, these blows aren't even necessarily direct shots to the head — certainly not always the most obvious or photogenic ones. They can also simply be body blows with such force and awkwardness that inertia causes the brain to slosh, unhinged, inside a skull more loosely containing it than we realized. Over time, the brain scars, in some cases even tearing at the stem.

Further lost in the polemical shuffle is the nuance that whereas known events such as brain bleeds or spinal cord injuries are discrete and acute, in numbers we can compile and debate over tradeoffs, CTE itself is a bit of a catch-all, elusive yet chronic. It remains a largely silent silo of harm, unprovable in individual cases prior to postmortem autopsy. Today some of the most committed researchers in the field are devising imaging techniques that might break through to a standard for detection of CTE in the living. They believe this will be a game-changer in the public debate.

Take it from me and don't bet on it. The industry's robust manufacture of doubt will always outpace the production of compelling but merely suggestive data. And the thing is, the scariest part of this story of our systematic national mental health debasement, with eyes wide open, are these very nuances.

So here I turn to the mission of enlightening a larger audience on another phenomenon, football conditioning deaths, with special moral urgency for those afflicting the non-professional and those so young that they don't even have legal agency. For purposes of this discussion, comprehensiveness is as unnecessary as it is unattainable. I've chosen to develop full narratives targeting three common associated etiologies: bronchial asthma, exertional sickling, and exertional heatstroke. But more important than the foreground facts (which, with all respect to the bereaved families, always seem much more alike than different) are their institutional backstories.

Transforming our grasp of how these stories are clusters, not isolated incidents, requires a sense of proportion lacking in the entertainment values of conventional coverage. While mulling whether football belongs in our public schools, we should consider that when you screw up the hire of an algebra teacher, you might momentarily impede the aspirations of a hungry learner — but when you screw up the hire of a football coach, you might wind up killing a kid and maiming many others.

Youth football conditioning deaths are annual events, like the turning of the colors of leaves. They can't faithfully be dismissed as outliers. They're given only piecemeal mention in local (and now and then national) media. Nonetheless, it's evident that every summer, like clockwork, several American boys perish simply from sloppily conceived or autocratically administered conditioning drills. Let's say it out loud and again: boys and young men are dropping dead on the spot, with regularity. These exercises in excess were putatively designed to get them in better shape for competition. Their more angular agenda, however, was to certify "toughness."

Like enemy-controlled villages in a murky war, kids are getting killed for their own good.

In many cases, the fallen athlete just loved the activity, we're told. Or his parents did — or at least they signed off on it. (The outsourcing of parenting to Svengali coaches is a major sports theme both in football harm, a phenomenon affecting mostly boys, and in widespread coach sexual abuse in individual Olympic sports like swimming and gymnastics, affecting mostly girls.)

My modest goal in exposing this morbid strain in the foreshortened lives of American males is to establish a pattern and to stir the movement to fix it. Adult authority and athletic standards shouldn't be so unregulated merely for the purpose of providing grist and a developmental infrastructure for professionalized mass spectacle. The unethical use of young human guinea pigs to fill out rosters below the $15-billion-or-so National Football League manifests not child growth, but adult exploitation at its most chilling.

In the end, wherever the locale or whatever the underlying medical cause, all youth football conditioning deaths are casualties of war, leaving behind grieving mothers, fathers, siblings, and communities. Decade after decade, we casually assume the legitimacy of this war on ourselves, undeclared and unannounced, without national purpose, waged in the domestic confines of a game — one whose militarized metaphor crosses the line. It's time to start challenging that assumption.

When the full history of football gets written, it may well come across, like slavery, bloody foreign adventures, or other more overt black marks, as a long and unchallenged chapter of American jihadism. Even if that specific image is considered exaggerated or inflammatory, the appraisal is not likely to be pretty. Most especially bothersome is the tortured relationship of African-Americans to football, which is said to provide the meritocracy often lacking in other realms of national life. But this opportunity fosters collusive semi-secrecy surrounding sickle cell trait–driven conditioning deaths, one of the key factors that will have commentators of the future wondering why Blacks at all economic levels came to love football, when football clearly didn't love them back. (See Agu, Ted, Chapters 2 through 4 below.)

Credit for catalyzing contemporary ideas for scaling back football goes to critics, researchers, and journalists better positioned and timelier than myself, many of whom placed themselves squarely inside the tradition of the American sports project. In the early years of this century, Alan Schwarz of the *New York Times* was the writer who crystallized for mass consumption the new information from autopsies of the brains of Mike Webster and other dead Pittsburgh Steelers players. Those studies were undertaken on the initiative of Dr. Bennet Omalu, a native Nigerian with scant connection to the NFL establishment, who at the time was the deputy coroner of Allegheny County, Pennsylvania. Shunned by top medical journals with NFL ties, Omalu was profiled in a magazine as a pioneer whistleblower, and ultimately portrayed by Will Smith in the 2015 movie *Concussion*. The film flopped, both at the box office and as a significant agent of change.

The orientation of my own reporting and analysis has been the economic and social ecosystem, the jockeying in the marketplace for commercial solutions, and the personal vanities of the figures who promoted them. I've tagged this demimonde "Concussion Inc." In their best-selling 2013 book, *League of Denial*, about the NFL's navigation of the post-Omalu period of exposure, explanation, and adaptation, authors Mark Fainaru-Wada and Steve Fainaru cited some of this area of work and even entitled one chapter "Concussion, Inc." (*sic*).

I had a minor friendship with Dr. Omalu — we once dined together near French Camp, California, where he was taking a lunch break from his duties at the time as chief medical examiner of San Joaquin County. Our friendship withered under scrutiny. Without a doubt, Omalu had been slighted in the attention given by the *Times*'s Schwarz and others to his estranged Boston-based research and advocacy partners, Dr. Robert Cantu and the former Harvard football player and WWE performer Chris Nowinski. Whether the main factor in these slights was racial bias, as Omalu complained, or simply the Ivy League elite bias of the Newspaper of

Record is debatable. I've never hesitated to criticize Cantu and Nowinski, especially when they accepted NFL money and were in my view compromised by it. But I also tried to call all the balls and strikes as I saw them.

Bennet Omalu, not quite as naive and disenfranchised as his cinematic persona sought to portray, had his own feet of clay. He insisted on bragging that he'd personally coined the term "chronic traumatic encephalopathy," when it was obvious it had been in the medical literature for nearly a century, to capture what lay people have called the "punch-drunk syndrome" of former boxers. It remains a mystery why Omalu didn't appreciate that such brand-hogging was counterproductive — that he would have been far more effective just acknowledging as much, placing his findings in the context of historical football harm denial, and settling for his due in the considerable achievement of locking broad public awareness for the first time onto the patent applicability of CTE to the football setting.

As Will Smith was failing to snare an Oscar nomination for *Concussion*, the movie's main producer, Ridley Scott, was setting up the Bennet Omalu Foundation. The University of Pittsburgh was an odd home for it, given that the medical center there was the Super Bowl champion corrupt cell of NFL doctors, paid deniers, and commercial exploiters. (One piece of quackery, the ImPACT "concussion management system," which is Pitt intellectual property, is widely peddled to high school football programs eager to demonstrate that they are doing "something" around public concern over the safety of the brains of teenagers.) But that was the least of the foundation's problems. The board of directors turned out to be stuffed with Scott's wife and movie-making pals and even Dr. Julian Bailes, the medical director for the little league organization Pop Warner Football. To anyone following the football safety debate, Bailes was notorious for his preposterously false claim of "no reported deaths" attributable to youth football in the 40 years before 2013. There were around 30 such deaths throughout that period. (Alec Baldwin portrayed Bailes in the movie.)

As for advocacy and activism, the Omalu Foundation did exactly nothing: it simply contracted with Scott's companies for website design and public relations services; published links to the same handful of news media articles found at multiple other sites (while, pointedly, censoring

Omalu's own powerful *New York Times* essay headlined "Don't Let Kids Play Football"); and promoted online donation buttons that, in the course of a year, yielded less than $3,000. After a series of articles at my website in 2016 exposing these defects, the foundation was abruptly shuttered.

In his song "American Pie," Don McLean pinpoints "the day the music died": February 3, 1959, when three early rock and roll luminaries went down together in a plane crash. In my own low-profile journey writing about football, it became no longer possible to consume the sport without a core cringe subsequent to October 22, 1989. That was the day I attended a game between the San Francisco 49ers and the New England Patriots at Stanford Stadium outside Palo Alto, California.

The backstory involves what I was doing there and why the game wasn't being played, per normal scheduling, at Candlestick Park in San Francisco. I was following Joe Montana, the 49ers quarterback, for a cover story for the *New York Times Magazine*. And the Loma Prieta earthquake, five days earlier, had forced Candlestick to be closed for repairs and the game to be relocated 30 miles south of its original planned site.

Though eventful for my career, the game itself was a trivial checked box on the football calendar. Under first-year head coach George Seifert, the juggernaut 49ers were en route to their second consecutive Super Bowl championship and fourth in nine years. Montana was in the midst of arguably the finest season of his Hall of Fame career. In the second quarter, he injured a knee on a hit in the pocket and was carted off. Backup Steve Young replaced him for the remainder of the game. (My main concern at the time was whether Montana had suffered a serious injury that would put him out of action for a lengthy period, jeopardizing my *Times Magazine* article. Turned out he was OK.) The 49ers pulled away in the second half, winning by a final score of 37–20.

I was unnerved by two sights.

The first was a play early in the game when a 49ers safety, a hard-hitting Texan named Jeff Fuller, took down the Patriots running back, John Stephens. Either Fuller used poor tackling technique by leading with his head instead of his shoulder — or, as participants and observers have come to articulate to a fare thee well, the speed and territorial demands of this sport simply don't allow the time for textbook form on every play, at least not if you want to succeed. In any event, the two players' helmets collided head-on. In the kind of aftermath serially captured in the 1975 dystopian movie *Rollerball*, Fuller was the one who didn't get up.

Bill Walsh, the 49ers' recently retired legendary coach, was doing commentary that day on the game's NBC broadcast. After viewing the replay, Walsh assessed the Fuller injury for the audience: "He's concussed."

Fuller was not concussed; he was partially paralyzed. Eventually most of the feeling in his body was restored, but he'd never play another down of football, nor ever again have full civilian use of his right arm. In the Stanford Stadium press box, I was sitting next to Dave Anderson, the *Times*'s Pulitzer Prize–winning columnist. Anderson borrowed my media guide so he could crib information about Fuller for a short side news article about football's latest casualty, to supplement his regular column sizing up the 49ers' steamroller progression to another championship.

The second disturbing sight related to the game's changed venue. On the fly, the 49ers' media relations staff had needed to redesign procedures, since the Stanford accommodations were different than those of Candlestick, and in particular the distance between the press box and the locker rooms was considerably greater. They decided to herd all the print media writers down from the press box and deposit them along the 49ers sideline with about five minutes left in the fourth quarter. This set us up for a quicker hop to the locker rooms for timely postgame interviews.

Had this been a basketball game, we would have labeled what I proceeded to witness at close range "garbage time" in a blowout. The outcome hadn't been in doubt for some time. In football, however, there's no such thing as garbage time; there's no playing at half-speed, even after the rout is on, since almost every block and tackle, by definition, has a baseline of violent contact, often from a peculiar angle. Moreover, regardless of the score, the first-string players almost always remain on the field. From the standpoint of those manning the offensive side's "skill positions" in particular — quarterback, running backs, pass receivers — their counting stats of yards gained on the ground or through the air still matter, and the ratios of targets, completions, and interceptions could still impact all-star team selections and the next contract negotiations. There's no incentive to hold back, regardless of the score. Indeed, according to the creed of these athletes, easing up can be the most dangerous formula of all for injury, as well — relaxing best practices might confuse muscle memory and leave you more vulnerable rather than less.

I'd seen NFL practices from sideline proximity on many occasions. I also had viewed football game action from this perspective, not merely through an antiseptic television lens or a remote seat, though at no higher than the high school level. This time, for some reason, watching the inexorable, primitive cycle of the gridiron play out in the meaningless last minutes of a one-sided game — snap the ball; the equivalent of half a dozen car crashes in a few seconds; huddle up and do it again — bothered me. The capper came when 49ers running back Roger Craig swept around the left end and into the usual chaotic pile out of bounds. This scrap heap of hulking male humanity landed perhaps seven feet away from me, and I wasn't in danger of being plowed over myself, as sideline photographers sometimes are. Still, the robotic pornography of the violence was unsettling in a way that, as a fan or journalist, I'd never before processed quite so intimately.

When the game ended, I did the sportswriter thing, meandering through the 49ers locker room, chatting with various players, looking for Joe Montana. (He was not around, having been carted off hours earlier for X-rays to confirm that no knee ligament was unduly stretched, no cartilage too severely torn, no meniscus irreversibly mangled.)

A tap on my shoulder and there was Mike Holmgren (later the Super Bowl–winning head coach for Brett Favre's Green Bay Packers) saying hello. My Montana story for the *Times Magazine* would be a breakdown of the craft of the quarterback position, not a conventional profile, and Holmgren, the 49ers' offensive coordinator, had given me more than an hour of his time a week earlier, on a morning before the start of practice in Santa Clara, to explain in detail just what it was about Montana's footwork, mechanics, and other attributes that stamped him as state of the art.

Shaking my head, I said to Holmgren, "That Jeff Fuller play — that was scary."

Holmgren replied, "They're all scary."

More than three decades later, that day continues to inform my views of where football is headed, whether quickly or slowly.

In the dialogue surrounding football and public health, we're well past the equivalent of those old warnings about tobacco. In the famous 1964 report, an advisory committee to the surgeon general found irrefutable causal links between cigarette smoking and mortality; between smoking and adverse birth outcomes; between smoking and emphysema, heart disease, and lung cancer. To some extent, our society has been engaged, in the ensuing half-century-plus, in the process of downsizing that industry, taking steps to limit its marketing and consumption, and trying to remain vigilant about technological offshoots such as vaping. Or at your most cynical, you might say we've been busy off-loading the ramifications of a multibillion-dollar global industry — alone exceeding the budgets of some developing nations — on both our own market's and the world's marginalized populations.

For football, the analogy of the surgeon general's report has been the episodes of public TBI, generally, and CTE, specifically, among the sport's elite athletes, past and present. Some fans have received this information with, at least, a civilized flinch (it's better than nothing, and it can influence degrees of fanaticism and patronage). One consequence is ambiguous evidence that football participation is in slow decline at the system's feeder levels, especially among the more socioeconomically privileged. In shorthand, the religion of football may remain as fervent as ever in rural Texas, *Friday Night Lights* land, while some high schools in better-off communities are starting to scramble to field full teams. Perhaps, in a bird's eye view later in the 21st century, we'll perceive the emergence of an explicit gladiator class, cut off from equitable access to society's other opportunities, and incentivized by fame and riches to make it their life's work to pursue a share of the profits in mass divertissement.

But here's the point about those masses: They're still there. They're not going away. Pro football's popularity continues to defy gravity. From television ratings for the games themselves to the ever-expanding content accessories of Super Bowl week (which long ago eclipsed Presidents' Day weekend as our de facto late winter national holiday), the numbers continue to go up, up, up — especially as the NFL grows savvier by the year in connecting its enterprise to musical acts and other corners of pop culture. Predictions of overexposure simply haven't been vindicated. The NFL now owns autumn Thursday nights as well as Sunday and Monday nights and the legacy Sunday afternoons, and has expanded live event venues to Mexico, England, and Germany. Friday nights are for the high schools. Saturday, from dawn in Honolulu, Hawaii, to midnight in Hampton, Virginia, offers those more narrowcasted yet grossly profitable TV bites of college action. And "action" is exactly the right word, as taboos and laws against gaming fall away and betting commerce gets mass-advertised.

Not very well processed is the extent to which supporting such a system from the bottom up requires massive public subsidies, most especially expenditures in our secondary schools and public fields, plus artificially underwritten line items of insurance and health care. In 2013, I attended something called a symposium on sports law and ethics sponsored by Santa Clara University in California. On one panel, in response to a question, the athletic director of Saint Francis High School in nearby Mountain View made the ridiculous assertion that his institution's high-powered football program had an annual budget of only $80,000. The accounting tricks required to transpose to the school's general funds the staff salaries, facilities maintenance, and insurance premiums of the football budget were apparent.

Such are the underpinnings of football world that critics and, eventually, policy-makers must focus on. Medical science was the basis of the *Concussion* movie, but the solution will not spring forth whole from any single critic's epiphany and earnestness. As in the case of the spiritual hold of a church, football is an institution in unnatural and inglorious burst prior to its decline. The only question is how long will be the tail of that decline, and how deadly will be the last flash of its lightbulb.

A campaign to curtail football and its carnage requires a multifaceted approach, one not limited to the sport's sexiest and most easily digested horror: that football kills the brain — preferably, that of a celebrity. Football also kills, period. It also maims — mentally, neurologically, orthopedically, and by destroying internal organs. It both ends lives and severely disfigures quality of life — individually, of course, but also collectively, in untold ways. Let's start telling and counting all of them.

When we home in on one facet — the several children a year who perish on American fields before they even have a chance to don helmets and shoulder pads — we begin to understand that these deaths aren't, at bottom, from bronchial asthma or exertional heatstroke or sickle cell trait attacks or coronary episodes. These are deaths *by football* — by a concededly wildly popular activity (and popular for some good reasons), freighted with a fundamentally obscene cost.

Football's "what price glory?" trope, a favorite of sentimental popular literature about it, needs to be taken across the board, in terms of its millions of participants, not just its few hundred most elite and hard-core. The last word belongs to a nation of spectators. Ameliorating the football problem is a task for all of us.

CHAPTER 1

Let's Go
to the
Videotape

Though they were just two places apart on the sprint line for the offensive and defensive backs, Jason Wright wasn't among the first teammates to see Rashidi Wheeler go down.

Not that Wright would have realized the extent of Wheeler's breathing difficulties this time, anyway. Like the other more than 60 Northwestern University football players participating in this conditioning drill (along with five high school recruits who were on hand illegally), Wright was used to seeing Rashidi's asthma attacks. In the first three years of his collegiate career he'd practiced and played through something like 30 of these episodes. Coordinating football and asthma management went back to Wheeler's days at Damien High School in La Verne, California, a Los Angeles County bedroom community. He routinely carried around an inhaler through which he'd take a quick whiff of albuterol, an anti-inflammatory corticosteroid, whenever he was in distress, including on the field. On August 3, 2001, huffing and puffing in sprint drills on a pitch ordinarily used for field hockey on Northwestern's Evanston, Illinois, campus near Lake Michigan, Rashidi clutched that inhaler in his fist.

Jason Wright, who was on the field with Wheeler, would go on to earn a psychology degree from Northwestern. Wright wasn't considered talented enough for selection in the NFL draft, but he had the determination to travel around to the auditions at scouting combines and tryout camps anyway. He wound up catching on as a free agent, and through much of a decade he found backup running back spots with the San Francisco 49ers, the Atlanta Falcons, the Cleveland Browns, and the Arizona Cardinals. Driven, educated, and organized, and a precocious leader, he became an NFL Players Association representative, or shop steward, during the 2011 owners' lockout. Wright went on to a career as an executive management consultant. Today he's president of the NFL's Washington Commanders.

The reason Wright at first didn't see what happened to Wheeler on that afternoon in 2001 was that Wright wasn't breathing so well himself — and it wasn't because of asthma.* At the point when Wheeler dropped to his hands and knees, gasping for air, the backs group had completed the first of four repetitions of 40-yard dashes — following ten reps at 100 yards, eight more at 80, and six at 60, with brief breaks in between. While Wheeler was being helped off the field, Wright tore into the last three of his own set of 40s.

Randy Walker, the head coach, had decreed that backs — such as Wheeler, a defensive safety, and Wright, a tailback / wide receiver and kick returner — had to run their 100s in under 14 seconds, their 80s in under 12, their 60s in under nine, and their 40s in under seven. Wright passed muster, but barely. At the conclusion of his final sprint — his 28th overall, covering a total of 2,160 yards, or about a mile and a quarter, over the course of around 12 minutes — he, too, collapsed.

Wheeler and Wright weren't alone. Between 4:30 and 5:00 p.m., as many as ten players slumped onto the artificial turf in states of disorientation. At least four of them needed medical attention: Wheeler, Wright, cornerback Raheem Covington, and running back Kevin Lawrence.

Nor did the spectacle of a bunch of burly, shirtless jocks dropping like flies shock anyone familiar with this most revered and despised ritual of

---

* Wright declined to be interviewed. This account combines interpretation of contemporaneous news coverage with independent reporting.

Coach Walker's infamously merciless workout regimen. Walker called the drill "the winning edge." He said the idea was to mirror a football game's quick bursts of action, alternating with pauses between plays for recovery. Northwestern had been a ferocious fourth-quarter come-from-behind team in 2000, and Walker credited this to their superior physical conditioning. And it was hard to argue with success. The Wildcats were defending Big Ten Conference co-champions. The media named Walker conference coach of the year. A national panel of peers honored him as Region 3 coach of the year.

One of the other players on the ground, along with Wheeler, was Pete Chapman, a 294-pound defensive tackle. Linemen weren't expected to run the drill as fast as the backs, but they had to complete the brutal cycle just the same. Any player at any position who failed to do so would have to retake the test two weeks hence in the truly oppressive heat of Kenosha, Wisconsin, site of Northwestern's formal preseason training camp. This was a prospect Chapman had particular cause to dread. The previous summer in Kenosha, during an end-of-practice series of 16 100-yard dashes, Chapman had been one of two players who passed out and were taken by ambulance to St. Catherine's Medical Center, where they were given intravenous fluids for dehydration. Now in Evanston, the temperature was 82 degrees Fahrenheit in moderate humidity, translating to a "heat index" of 87. Bothered by a sinus infection, Chapman was crumbling again.

Head athletic trainer Tory Aggeler and five members of his staff scrambled to administer first aid to all the fallen players. Larry Lilja, the director of strength and conditioning, and his assistant Tom Christian continued supervising the sprints. Lilja paced the sideline, barking out times and noting them on a clipboard. Christian operated the two video cameras recording the activities for later review by Walker and the whole coaching staff.

Fortunately for Jason Wright, his body refrained from shutting down until after he'd finished conquering "the winning edge." Staggering across the finish line, he lost consciousness and his body went into convulsions. When he regained his senses, he vomited. Amidst the dizziness and nausea, though, he'd remember feeling "as happy as I've ever been." He'd done it.

Now, in Kenosha, he could concentrate on skills work and securing a spot in the Wildcats' starting lineup.

Wright's moment of private exultation didn't last long. Near the bench on the sideline, he could make out some kind of commotion. Through blurred vision, he spotted a figure on the ground, a trainer bent over him. Moving closer, he saw that it was Rashidi Wheeler.

Wright heard someone say, "Rashidi lost his pulse."

On the videotape, Wheeler isn't the focus; he's just another guy laboring under the stress of the "the winning edge." By the time the backs hit their 60-yard sets, he's lagging seriously behind. On his first 60, he crosses the finish line right at the nine-second threshold. On his sixth and last 60, he's ten yards behind the pack. On his first 40, he's not even in the picture until after several teammates, who have already finished, turn around and yell encouragement: "Come on, Shidi!" . . . "Let's go, Shidi!" . . . "Keep moving!"

At 4:40 p.m., Wheeler sank to the ground. The others on their runs had to navigate around him. Wheeler's friend, linebacker Kevin Bentley, helped him up. Trainer Aggeler came over to assist. At first Wheeler insisted he was OK and could finish the drill, but then he let Bentley and Aggeler lead him to the bench on the sideline.

Between gasps, Wheeler complained, "I want to stop breathing."

Aggeler tried to get Wheeler to use his inhaler, but Rashidi was in too much distress to suck up the albuterol. Suspecting hyperventilation, Aggeler modeled slower breathing and instructed Wheeler to mimic him. Overall, the situation seemed under control, not "emergent," in athletic trainers' jargon. In fact, on the other side of the field, Kevin Lawrence looked to be in worse shape and in need of the head trainer's immediate attention. Aggeler ordered Mike Rose, a student training intern, to take over watching Wheeler.

Rose gave Wheeler a paper bag to breathe into. Exhaling carbon dioxide into an enclosed space is a common corrective for someone hyperventilating, but this bag had a hole in it. In any case, hyperventilation was starting to look like a misdiagnosis. Wheeler was saying it hurt to breathe. He said he wanted to lie down. He told Bentley, "K.B., I'm dying." The concerned people gathered around him weren't sure whether to take that remark literally. They thought not.

Ten minutes later, Wheeler fell off the bench and stopped breathing. Rushing over, Aggeler performed cardiopulmonary resuscitation. Wheeler didn't respond.

Aggeler shouted to an assistant to call 911. It was the early era of cell phones and none was readily available. The closest land line was a pay phone a few yards away, outside the field house of the Sports and Aquatic Center. That phone turned out to be out of order. Several players had their mobiles with them. Aggeler grabbed one and punched in 911. It took two tries to get connected. There was confusion at the Evanston dispatch center. A follow-up call from Northwestern's director of football operations, Justin Chabot, directed emergency units to the corner of Sheridan Road and Lincoln Street.

> *The video shows a surreal mix of chaos and business as usual. In the foreground, frantic personnel dart in front of the camera from one or the other direction. The final footage before the camcorders were shut off captures four players — Wright, Bentley, Covington, and Chasda Martin — kneeling in prayer a few feet from the paramedics working on Wheeler, and the ambulance rolling up and speeding away.*
>
> *In the background, the sprint drills proceed.*

Paramedics arrived on a fire truck at 5:09. Walker, the head football coach, wasn't at the drills; he was doing yard work at his home nearby. Alerted, Walker reached the field simultaneously with the ambulance, at 5:11. A group of ten of his players joined Walker in a caravan of cars behind the ambulance to Evanston Hospital, three minutes away.

Trainer Aggeler went, too — but not before interrogating several other players. They admitted to him that, before the workout, Wheeler was one of a group who had ingested doses of Ultimate Punch and Xenadrine, two over-the-counter nutritional supplements, from the family of ephedra stimulants that were banned by the National Collegiate Athletic Association. Aggeler grabbed samples of the supplements from the locker room, turned them over to the police gathering information for their report, and headed to the hospital.

The ambulance pulled up at 5:25. The emergency room resident, Dr. Morris Kharasch, could detect neither pulse nor respiration. A defibrillator was attached to Wheeler's chest. For 20 minutes, advanced cardiac life support was administered. It was useless.

One of the cell phones on the field was Wheeler's; Bentley had taken custody of it during the hospital vigil. Now the phone was used to relay the grim news to Rashidi's father, George Wheeler, a financial planner, who happened to be driving to Chicago along with his sister.

As soon as that conversation ended, the phone rang. It was Rashidi's mother, who worked for the California prison system. Oblivious to the drama of the last hour, she was just saying hello and checking in.

Thus it fell to Kevin Bentley the task of informing Linda Addison Will that her 22-year-old son had just dropped dead during an offseason football practice — without helmets or shoulder pads, or logic or humanity.

Rashidi Wheeler's death shook his family, his teammates, his university, and, ever so briefly, the sports world and the nation. Athletes are not supposed to die young; they are especially not supposed to die young as a result of the very things they do to stay in shape and compete as athletes. During the week of the Wheeler tragedy, three other football players across the country also died suddenly in non-contact drills. At the top of the list was Korey Stringer, a mountainous offensive lineman for the NFL's Minnesota Vikings, a victim of exertional heatstroke.

Taken together, these fatalities seemed to define an epidemiological cluster and to provide a frame for a broad discussion of extreme football coaching methods and the price paid by stars and would-be stars in their quest for fame and glory. Commentators pontificated on this theme for about three news cycles, encompassing the funeral, the emotional ceremony at which Wheeler's uniform number 30 was retired, and the speculation as to whether the Wildcats' 2001 season would proceed to go down the tubes in the wake of this "distraction." Soon, bread and circuses resumed. Rashidi Wheeler was a footnote — a casualty of a sport that draws its imagery from warfare. Whether the casualty was truly avoidable could be debated. Whether it was truly rare could not.

Closely examined, three elements converge to make the Rashidi Wheeler case something more than just a casual byproduct of fun and games.

The crucial first factor is the unique nature of the institution where he played college football and, perhaps only incidentally, was enrolled as a sociology major. Throughout its history, Northwestern University hadn't been a conventional college football factory. Over the years, the public has come to associate football-first excesses at places like the University of Alabama, whose late legendary coach, Bear Bryant, was depicted in a hagiographic film biography on ESPN that included unflattering accounts of his own sadistic practice sessions.* Or maybe the University of Nebraska, where a significant percentage of the state's population decks out in school colors and identifies with the fortunes of their Cornhuskers, the only major sports franchise in the area — notwithstanding their heroes' serial appearances on police blotters. Maybe these things are supposed to happen at public universities designed to pander to the rabblement. But they're not, in the name of Nobel, supposed to happen at Northwestern, which is recognized as one of the country's leading private research universities, regularly in the top ten of the *U.S. News & World Report* ratings of undergraduate programs, and with highly touted graduate and professional schools.

Moreover, not even Alabama or Nebraska, though touched by scandal of other kinds, ever lost a football player, let alone under such grotesque circumstances. At least part of the explanation of the Wheeler incident involves randomness. But, additionally, there was a key component of football death: big-time *aspiration*. This is the element adding fatal toxicity to the poisonous pressures felt by those already in the state of realization of success and feeling the pressure to maintain it. Northwestern's model

---

* The 1999 book *The Junction Boys*, by Jim Dent, is an account of a practice regime Bryant directed at a wilderness camp in Junction, Texas, for his 1954 Texas A&M team, before he went on to six national championships and legendary status at Alabama.

wasn't that of a football factory, but of a hybrid achiever. This group also includes universities such as Duke and Stanford, which likewise blend high academic standards with major team sports athletic success.

The problem in 2001 was that because Northwestern lacked Duke or Stanford's history of excellence in a particular high-revenue sport (football or men's basketball), the exigencies of the contemporary sports sweepstakes had sent it flying off the moral rails. The process began in earnest with the 1992 hire of head football coach Gary Barnett, an assistant at Colorado University. Three years later the Wildcats — representing the only private school in the Big Ten — came out of nowhere to make their first Rose Bowl appearance in nearly half a century.

In 1999, with a second conference title on his resume, Barnett jumped back to Colorado as head coach there for lots more money. Northwestern hired as his replacement Randy Walker, who had enjoyed an impressive run at Miami University in Ohio. Walker's mandate was to keep winning. And one manifestation of that mandate was loose oversight. A university administration suddenly drunk on sports revenue and attention seldom knows everything going on at its athletic department — or wants to know.

The second factor giving the Rashidi Wheeler story resonance is the complicated relationship between sports and race. Wheeler, like a majority of college athletes in the high-revenue sports, was African-American. The exploitation of jocks under this system is inextricably entwined with the national conversation on matters black and white. Within days of Rashidi's death, the Reverend Jesse Jackson, the civil rights leader, was counseling the Wheeler family and issuing pronouncements about this scenario's implications for the original sin of the American experience. Before long, with all the predictability of a pass on third-and-long, the race card was joined to the authority of the legal system by the arrival on the scene of Johnnie Cochran, the celebrated trial lawyer. Where reconciliation dialogues go to die, adversarial torts rarely fear to tread.

So here, finally and decisively, there were civil litigation forensics, that *sine qua non* of racial politics. A wrongful death lawsuit was the only, feeble way to exert justice. And the evidentiary tools included that crucial element of postmodern self-reference: the videotape smoking gun.

The precise cause of Wheeler's death was ambiguous — could it be attributed only to an exercise-induced bronchial asthma attack, as the coroner found? Or was Wheeler's use of borderline nutritional supplements the sole or at least a contributory cause, as the university would claim in its scorched-earth legal defense?

Regardless of the cause, the tape of the fateful practice session became a damning exhibit of college football's general callousness and sick priorities. The sights of inadequate medical personnel and resources at a borderline-illegal boot camp, and of drills forging ahead even as a dead or dying player was being carted away, combined to create what was nothing short of the sports world's counterpart to Rodney King, the African-American criminal suspect whose brutal beating by Los Angeles police officers was captured on tape in 1991 — officially opening the era of viral slam-dunk video in charged police interactions with minority suspects or innocent bystanders.

You may be asking, why was there a videotape of the "winning edge" sprint drills in the first place? The answer to that question goes to core characteristics of the prototype modern ultra-industrial, detail-obsessed, authoritarian-control-freak-run college football program. They were the third element making Rashidi Wheeler's death documented news at the time, and able to serve as documented history today.

This video was a production of the assistant coaches. Under NCAA rules, head coach Walker wasn't allowed to attend this offseason conditioning session. Indeed, under those same rules at that time, a football practice as early as August 3 also couldn't be either considered "mandatory" or kept on the official books. However, the word came down to the players, via Walker's staff, that universal participation was . . . *highly encouraged*. The truth is that in a big-bucks enterprise that's now a 365-day-a-year operation, the distinction between voluntary and mandatory has been pulverized like a quarterback by a blind-side blitz.

Videotaping ensured a crude record of who attended the session and who skipped it, who was in shape pre–training camp and who wasn't.

Under the same wink-wink rules, head coaches aren't allowed to supervise a "voluntary" workout. A nice videotape, however, could memorialize the event and reinforce written reports from assistants on who showed up and who slacked off, who was a man and who was a wimp. Generally, video is that indispensable tool of modern coaching. It's used to study technique and to break down opposing teams' tendencies. Nowadays every major coaching staff has one or more full-time positions, known as "quality control," dedicated to coordinating video production, editing, and study.

The Rashidi Wheeler tape would reveal a good deal about another kind of quality control. For, intentionally or not, this video helped establish that eight trainers and strength and conditioning staffers were indeed on hand that day — with roles obviously oriented more toward serving Randy Walker's win-at-all-cost agenda than the health and well-being of their charges. (Depositions later would confirm that Rick Taylor, the university's athletic director, was also watching the drill from the periphery, along with Chabot, the university official who placed one of the 911 calls.)

After an internal investigation, Northwestern conceded it had committed a technical violation of NCAA rules. An illegally scheduled mandatory practice is a so-called secondary infraction, meaning it's not considered something that gives the offending team a direct competitive advantage. With the support of the NCAA, the university announced it was self-imposing a proportionate sanction: as penance, the Wildcats football team forfeited the right to stage six regular practices.

"Six practices!" Rashidi's mother, Linda Will, said to me in our lone conversation on the phone in late 2001. "That's the value Northwestern placed on my son's life."*

Someone with a perspective not freighted with a mother's grief might note that the value of Rashidi Wheeler's life also would be imperfectly monetized in the family's subsequent lawsuit for wrongful death. Still, at the level of metaphor, there's no denying the accuracy of Will's equation and its moral implications.

About that financial settlement . . . Will wanted no part of it. What she wanted from Northwestern was her day in court. And if there were to be

---

* Johnnie Cochran's law office, which had given me (and other journalists) a VHS copy of the videotape it had acquired of the sprint drill, later tried, on Will's instructions, to get me to return it.

a settlement, she had one non-negotiable and non-financial provision: the firing of Randy Walker.

Will wound up getting neither her day in court nor her non-financial provision. Legal restitution for her son's death became mixed up with the full package of post-divorce conflicts between Linda Will and George Wheeler; and any lawyer will tell you that an aggressive litigation strategy is only as strong as its weakest link. In August 2005, Cook County Judge Kathy Flanagan denied Will's request to continue the case. For all practical purposes, the court shoved down a grieving mother's throat a settlement that was agreeable to the other parties. The next month the figure was finalized: $16 million. Having written off its latest cost of doing business, football world turned the page.

Northwestern, of course, didn't fire Randy Walker. In April 2006, the university gave him a two-year contract extension.

Two months later, on June 29, Walker suffered a heart attack and died. He was 52.

CHAPTER 2

Death by Sickling. What's That?

ounded in 1868 as one of the first great land-grant institutions of higher learning, the University of California at Berkeley today is probably the world's most famous public university. Its history of highlights runs the gamut from that 1964 culture war flashpoint, the Free Speech Movement, to the invention of the cyclotron particle accelerator by Professor Ernest O. Lawrence, to the development of the first flu vaccine. Cal* boasts record numbers of Nobel Laureates and MacArthur Foundation "genius award" winners. Earl Warren, the chief justice for Supreme Court cases ending racial segregation and implementing many other historic reforms, got his law school education at Berkeley. The school's motto is *"Fiat Lux"* ("Let light be made").

At Memorial Stadium, the football field on the eastern edge of campus, there is now displayed a plaque with these words:

---

* As used here, "Cal" and "UC-Berkeley" are interchangeable. Cal is the flagship of the University of California system. The university system as a whole is referred to as "UC."

FOREVER IN OUR HEARTS

Ted Obinna Agu

May 8, 1992 – February 7, 2014

LOVED BY ALL

Beloved Son, Brother and Friend

We Miss You

Agu died in a bizarre extreme conditioning drill. American males Agu's age and younger expire every year under broadly similar conditions. What perhaps most distinguishes Agu's death is that in Berkeley, a place celebrated for studying the world and the human condition in multiple academic disciplines, the university deployed the playbook of football world to execute a brazen cover-up of the circumstances. And as we'll see, that cover-up largely succeeded.

All kinds of claims can be advanced for the net positives of the University of California. Some of them are so: collective undergraduate enrollment at statewide campuses, totaling nearly a quarter of a million students, ranks it third behind the California State University and State University of New York systems in terms of number of college graduates turned out annually.[*] But there's no dodging the uncomfortable truth that, in its wedding to the football industry, this institution might as well be a cigarette company or a gun manufacturer. Instead of *Fiat Lux* in the story of an avoidable death — indeed, arguably, an unindicted manslaughter — the university produced *Lux Impediatur*: "Let light be blocked."

In labeling the cover-up brazen, I don't mean to imply that it was also, necessarily, off the charts by the standards of corporate reputational and legal defense tactics. Indeed, what makes Cal's avoidance of accountability most worth in-depth analysis is its very routineness. To be sure, this task required vigilance, effort, and paperwork by the university's employed protectors (or maybe it was ensuring the most limited traces of paperwork). But that's what bureaucrats are paid to do every day. If you expected agencies

---

[*] California State University campuses offer only undergraduate degrees and are not to be confused with UC.

of inquiry, such as the campus police or the California Public Records Act compliance office, to register an honorable measure of independence or to facilitate the harshest scrutiny or criticism, you were mistaken.

The cover-up, as the term is so advisedly used here, was evident from the opening moments. Scott Anderson, then the head football athletic trainer at the University of Oklahoma (now retired but still a leading critic of conditioning drill excesses and an active monitor of the deaths from them), has a network of sources at football programs across the country.[*] On the morning of February 7, 2014, one of them told Anderson of having just spoken with a Cal assistant coach, who was expressing the fears of almost everyone at the Berkeley football complex's Simpson Center for Student-Athlete High Performance with regard to the fatality that had just occurred.

"It's a sickle cell death," the assistant coach said flatly to Anderson's source.[**]

An article with educated speculation that a Golden Bears player had succumbed to an exertional attack associated with sickle cell trait — a syndrome I'll proceed to explain — quickly got posted on the front page of the website of CBS Sports. In addition to challenging the lethargy of its audience with respect to football harm, the report, had it ever gotten off the ground, would have been up against the problem of public confusion as to the distinctions between *sickle cell trait*, a genetic marker, and the much better known *sickle cell anemia*. The latter, a disease, is an acute, disablingly painful, and ultimately often fatal red blood cell disorder. There are high-profile campaigns around consciousness-raising about sickle cell

---

[*] Chapter 8 below has more on the work of Anderson and his colleague, retired University of Oklahoma football team physician Dr. Randy Eichner, to document and raise awareness of football conditioning drill deaths and their causes.

[**] Scott Anderson has not named those in his chain of sources. From independent reporting, I'm all but certain of the identity of the assistant coach. The day after the Agu death, that coach was known to be telling friends that top university officials thought the cause was exertional sickling but were "hoping against hope" that it would be found to be standard cardiac arrest. The coach, now on the staff of a program in another region of the country and at a lower subdivision of the NCAA football hierarchy, didn't respond when I reached out to him. I'm not naming the coach here out of respect for Anderson's own sources and methods.

disease, with fundraising pegged to the search for a cure. (As this book was being published, there was a breakthrough in gene therapy that shows promise for being curative.)

Sickle cell trait is something different: a genetic condition carried by one in 12 African-Americans. There are perhaps three million total carriers in the U.S. It's a more complicated phenomenon, sociologically as well as medically.*

First and foremost, the trait is an important data point for prospective parents: if both the father and the mother are carriers, then the risk that their children will be afflicted with sickle cell anemia is substantially elevated. Mere trait carriers themselves, however, can lead essentially normal lives. Again, the trait is a condition, not a full-blown disease.

But the trait has an associated caveat: carriers must be attentive to the possible onset of sudden attacks during extreme exercise. The medical literature calls these episodes exertional sickling, or ES. If ES occurs and gets detected in a timely fashion and the victim stops what he was doing, then everything usually turns out OK. But if the victim and his handlers regard what is happening as a garden-variety workout challenge, one to push through instead of to respect by bringing to a halt, then the worst consequences can play out in deadly minutes.

The prevalent medical explanation of what occurs during ES is "explosive rhabdomyolysis." This is a result of a carrier's stiffer and stickier red blood cells. These cells proceed to logjam the flow of blood. In "rhabdo," dead muscle tissue breaks down and enters the bloodstream, poisoning it. Within a short time, in the best cases, the victim can suffer severe liver damage. In the worst cases, he dies.

While ES deaths are relatively sudden, their timeline differs from that of heart attacks, in the sense that they play out in stages, rather than all at once. That's why vigilance is so important, and why it's possible to tease out ES as an underreported subset of football conditioning deaths. If a victim carries the trait and those around him know as much yet don't

---

* The trait is also associated with malaria, and hence is seen in 0.5 percent of Hispanics, as well as in small numbers of Mediterraneans, Middle Easterners, Indians, and whites.

take appropriate steps at the onset of ES, then they might as well not have known at all.

On the platform of the football industry and its African-American-heavy athlete base, deaths by ES during conditioning drills are both less random and more morally objectionable than deaths by heart disease. What Cal did to Ted Agu was sloppy, uncaring, and unbecoming. No matter how academically esteemed a university might be, when it takes the plunge into the multibillion-dollar industry of intercollegiate athletics, such a school inevitably finds itself positioned at just another way station on the road to extracurricular outrage and scandal.

Ways to contain scandal include keeping general awareness low and completely disclaiming direct awareness when the worst happens. In football world, growing consciousness of the sickling attack problem is slowed by a central feature of American life: the limited range of opportunities Black men are perceived to enjoy, and indeed actually enjoy. In our society, two of the areas probably operating closest in accordance with the ideals of a true meritocracy are the military and sports; there, it seems to matter more than almost anywhere else not who you know or where you came from — only how well you can perform. Not coincidentally, these also have become settings where poorly regulated conditioning programs trigger excess deaths of Black males on an annual basis. African-Americans die disproportionately in military basic training boot camps, as well as in football conditioning drills. Some of these deaths are from ES, whether or not so listed, at the time of death or ever. A 1987 Army study found that Black recruits with sickle cell trait were 30 times likelier to die during basic combat training than those without the trait. Police and fire recruits face similar challenges. (Trait carriers also need to be alert in activities such as mountain climbing, scuba diving, and riding in airplanes without pressurized cabins.)

Outside of football, the weirdness of the political dynamics of ES are most evident in controversies over police brutality toward Black suspects and criminals. The literature identifies the occasional ES case of someone fleeing law enforcement officers. But perhaps most perversely, defendant police in George Floyd–like cases, in which a suspect was pinned down with a knee to the neck or held in a lethal chokehold, sometimes send up a speculative flare that it was actually an instance of ES, beyond the control of the arresting officer.

Getting back to the context of an educational institution's legal exposure, the warps in understanding sickle cell trait get measured in the number of digits following a dollar sign when inevitable lawsuits reach inevitable settlements.

The CBSSports.com coverage of the Ted Agu death on February 7, 2014, was the only version containing the truth that Agu had not had a generic coronary episode but, rather, expired from ES. This was information with the potential to galvanize public understanding of one of sports' most insidious and least acknowledged killers. Thanks to the cowardice of various parties, such understanding never came close to fruition. Within hours after the article went up online, it was taken down, in a sequence both little noticed by readers and never explained by CBS Sports. (CBS didn't respond to my multiple requests for comment on how and why the piece got pulled.)

Insurance companies were invented for the occasional sketchy and litigated death. It's a cost of business. From the first moments after Agu expired, Cal knew that it would be entangled not just in a defense in court but also in a larger and more image-urgent campaign engaging teams of lawyers and public relations stage managers. The key question became whether the university could bury significant general public knowledge of the cause of death here, which was ES. At the very least through the crucial period of first impression, could they succeed in ascribing the event to another, purportedly unavoidable, act of God?

In the fundamentals, Ted Agu's is the tragedy of the death of an athlete too young. The Agu meta-story is something more: the manipulations of the flagship public university in the nation's most populous state to dodge reflection and accountability. In this mission, Cal was enabled by the self-censorship of CBS Sports, and later would be enabled by the similar behavior of other mainstream news outlets, most notably the *San Francisco Chronicle*.

———

If you were searching for a central casting exhibit of a student-athlete who was in football purely for love of the game, Ted Agu was your guy. His parents were Nigerian immigrants. Ted came out of Frontier High School in Bakersfield, with a body type somewhere between a linebacker and a defensive lineman. This made him a very good player but not an elite one; he was neither quite bulky enough to play on the line at the NCAA Division I level nor quite fast enough to play behind it. As a result, he didn't attract a scholarship offer. But he had a passion to attend Berkeley, where he got accepted and became a pre-med major, and he had a passion for football. It all added up to that most amateur of amateurs in college football: the non-scholarship or "walk-on" squad member.

Now that the NCAA has grudgingly acknowledged things like the annual fluid transfer between schools of free agent players and the rights of student-athletes to profit from their celebrity (even if still not to be directly salaried), college football has taken a major step toward making the talent professionals, in all but name. In this environment, walk-ons have always been inconvenient accessories at best, annoyances at worst. Under the rules, they cannot be summarily turned away, so long as they show up and do everything asked of them. This is all bound up in the useful fiction that a university's money-driven sports team is actually an educational asset, not just a commercial brand. In most athletic conferences, all eligible players are allowed to dress in uniform and be on the sidelines at home games, though no more than 80 can actually see action in the game. For visiting games, a total of only 70 can travel.

With rare exception, walk-ons are part of the "non-travel" portion of the team. Non-travelers include "red shirts," scholarship players who are considered to have potential to be contributors to the main squad but are being held back because of injuries or for other developmental reasons. In this way, they can retain a year of their athletic eligibility while attending school (or at least going through the motions of same). Other non-travelers are just long-shot scrubs, including the walk-ons.

At many programs, the non-travel group gets subjected to the harshest extra drills. Part of the idea is that, as understudies, they need to push themselves even harder to improve. Another part is that they can be driven into the ground without the fear of losing playing time to injury, since they had none in the first place. A third part — also central to the psychology that the sport is a war and that the practice for it has the same stakes as training for the Green Berets or the Navy SEALs — applies specifically to the walk-ons: no one on the coaching staff sheds a tear if an extra-punishing regimen turns out to induce a hanger-on to give up, walk away, and stop taking up locker room space and other team resources.

Ted Agu was no quitter. By 2014, he was in his fourth and final year. He was universally respected by teammates, including and maybe especially by the scholarship athletes among them. Free ride through college or not, Agu was a natural leader. Faced with the harshest demands on the field and in the study hall sessions off it, he led by example, motivating others to give 100 percent too. He liked to party, but he also put in hours at the library to support good grades. One of Agu's best friends was a more talented defensive lineman, Ernest Owusu, also a son of African immigrants. After his Cal career, Owusu briefly made the rosters of teams in the Canadian Football League and the NFL (only the provisional "taxi squads" there), before returning to Berkeley, settling into a marketing job, and marrying the school's beach volleyball coach. (Owusu, a sickle cell trait carrier like Agu, also once had a scary bout with ES and later spoke out about it.)

Then there was Agu's conditioning level. One teammate called him "a fit monster." He was always the one out in front of the other linemen in exercises. When these were running drills, he often would find his fellow "bigs" too slow and decide to run off with the linebackers or the backfield players. He was equally impressive in the weight room; another teammate recalled watching the 250-pound Agu do a squat lift of 525 pounds. In sum, if you didn't know that Agu was a sickle cell trait carrier, with unique risks calling for extra levels of vigilance, then you would have marked him as last on the list of players who might die in a drill.

Agu *was* a trait carrier. And the university and its coaching, training, and medical staffs knew as much, since he'd opted into the NCAA's voluntary sickle cell trait screening program, which was enacted in 2010, and tested positive. Agu was one of at least three known trait carriers on the team. What would happen to him therefore raised the uncomfortable larger question of exactly how major college football programs accommodate the presence of these trait carriers in the operation of their conditioning programs.

In Agu's case, we know only that when the worst happened, Cal seemed to do nothing to take his risk into account. We further know that the university triggered massive fact-massaging resources toward concealing the truth.

In November 2012, Cal fired Jeff Tedford, the head football coach. Tedford had been there for 11 seasons, and the early ones had been successful, thanks to his golden touch with developing quarterbacks, including a guy named Aaron Rodgers. But the Golden Bears had gone into decline in recent years. When they won only three games in '12, a change was ordered.

The new head coach was Daniel "Sonny" Dykes. Son of the former Texas Tech head coach William "Spike" Dykes, Sonny was a rising star in college coaching. For five years he worked under his father's successor at Texas Tech, Mike Leach, who was credited with inventing a fast-paced offensive scheme called the Air Raid. Dykes went on to stints as offensive coordinator at Arizona and head coach at Louisiana Tech.

The deal for Dykes at Cal guaranteed him $9.7 million across five years. In 2016, two years after Ted Agu died on his watch, the coaching carousel rumor mill put out the word that Dykes was being wooed for other head coaching opportunities. Often such rumors are generated by the "highly sought after" coach's agents or surrogates. Cal responded by tearing up Dykes's existing contract with two years remaining, and signing him to an extension, through 2019 — raising his annual base pay from $2.3 million to $2.525 million, and throwing in performance incentive bonuses of up to $600,000 per.

That didn't work out so well, and by 2018 Dykes was out at Cal. He returned to his native Texas as head coach at Southern Methodist University in Dallas. In 2019, Dykes was a finalist for the Football Writers Association of America's Eddie Robinson Coach of the Year Award. In 2022, he jumped to SMU's rival, Texas Christian University in Fort Worth, and immediately won a surprise berth in the national championship game won the following January by Georgia. Dykes became the hands-down coach of the year.[*]

Dykes was just one of the several Cal football and sports department luminaries, directly or indirectly implicated in Agu's death, who would suffer no career consequences. Almost without exception, every central figure of the story, like Dykes, "fell upward" to better jobs.

At Berkeley, one of Dykes's first moves was to bring in his own strength and conditioning assistant from Louisiana Tech. His name was Damon Harrington. He replaced Mike Blasquez, who had been at Cal for 11 years, the last two with the football program. Harrington didn't appear to have undergone an interview for the job nor, for that matter, to have gone through any of the procedures of a formal job posting and vetting of a pool of candidates; he was simply installed on prerogative of the new head coach. Cal paid Harrington $150,000 a year. His contract included an $8,000 incentive bonus if the team placed in a postseason bowl game.

Harrington's stated job was to get Dykes's players in shape. But as in any regime change, there was a second and more important, if only implicit, role: "culture change." Jeff Tedford's last several teams had been regarded as not just underperforming but soft — the worst insult that could be leveled at a football team. Under Blasquez — as players later testified in the Agu family's lawsuit — the emphasis of the strength and conditioning program had been on technique in the weight room, the better to build bulk wedded to flexibility. Harrington, the new sheriff in town, brought a different approach.

One player said that whereas Blasquez "wanted to make you a better athlete," Harrington was all about "some down south mental toughness. 'We're building some soldiers here,'" he would say.

---

[*] After the championship game, Dykes prepared to build for even better things in 2023–24 by hiring Kendal Briles as offensive coordinator. While on the football staff at Baylor University the previous decade under his father, head coach Art Briles, Kendal Briles had helped cover up campus rapes by football players. According to a 2017 lawsuit against Baylor, the younger Briles implemented what was called a "show 'em a good time" approach with recruits. Specifically, the assistant coach took top high school players who were considering Baylor to strip clubs and made women in the university's "hostess program" available for sex.

Another player testified that Harrington's philosophy was "it doesn't matter about speed, doesn't matter about strength. Only matters about toughness. . . . So a lot of the stuff he does is to make us, in his words, 'tough as shit.'"

From the coach's Twitter account, he promoted a philosophy of max effort at all times, and, to boot, being a little crazy about it. Accompanying some of the tweets were things like images of the actor Russell Crowe from the movie *Gladiator*. Nor did Harrington mind extending his fantasy projections to the motivational rhetorical buttons of vulgarity or homophobia. Stanford University was Cal's traditional regional rival. When he perceived a lack of effort from his charges, Harrington's words of inspiration were: "Stanford has their cock in our ass!"

As expected, Harrington was especially hard on the non-travel group in Thursday morning workouts. He called this crew his "Crusaders."

On Thursday, October 31, 2013, Harrington scheduled a conditioning drill session for the non-travel group. At least one player wasn't there. Accounts differ as to why Fabiano Hale, a freshman running back, skipped the practice. In one version, Hale was doing extra studying for a test the next day. In another version, he just decided to take the day off for Halloween.

In any event, the conditioning coach told his gathered non-travel players that he wasn't pleased. His immediate response was collective punishment. That day Harrington doubled and tripled down on his sets of the always brutal conditioning drill. There were extras of "up-downs," in which you run in place, and on orders, plop to the ground on your belly and pop right back up for more running. Harrington piled on, especially, with an exercise called the "bear crawl." This has nothing to do with Cal's mascot, the golden bear. In the bear crawl, you go to the ground on all fours and lunge across a distance in incremental hand-and-foot steps, first one side then the other. This day the non-travel group was ordered to do bear crawls, over and over and over. Harrington seemed not satisfied until enough of them were vomiting into the turf.

Afterward, Harrington brought his athletes together. Noting the unexcused absence of one teammate, he said it was not his job to punish any individual for not showing up. The responsibility for that, the coach said, belonged to his peers. They were the ones who needed to take care of this situation, make sure everyone among them was accountable.

"By any means necessary," Harrington added, slamming his fist into his other, open palm for emphasis.

Late in the afternoon the next day, Fabiano Hale walked through the door of the locker room at the Simpson Center. He was met with a punch, either from behind or on his half-blind side, by J.D. Hinnant, a 260-pound freshman offensive tackle. The blow caused a three-inch laceration on Hale's right ear and soft-tissue swelling on the back of his head. If Hale wasn't already unconscious when he fell to the floor, Hinnant finished the job with additional punches and kicks.

It was a scene of a "code red" criminal assault by an underling who had been goaded by the suggestive language of an authority figure — something straight out of *A Few Good Men*, Rob Reiner's movie based on Aaron Sorkin's play, a legal thriller about the court-martial of two Marines who murdered a fellow service member for falling short of their demanding standards.

A woozy Hale wandered into the equipment room. Teammates noticed that his behavior was abnormal, and they summoned the team physician, Dr. Casey Batten, who sent Hale to the campus health services clinic, the Tang Center. From there he was transported to the emergency room of Berkeley's Alta Bates Medical Center, where he'd remain overnight.

Hale's parents, near Santa Cruz 75 miles to the south, got a phone call from a friend who was a parent of a teammate. They were told that Fabiano was in the hospital after being brutally attacked. A flurry of text messages confirmed the name of the assailant and the fact that, as one text put it, Hinnant was "upset because the coach made the team work extra hard in practice because Fabiano didn't show up." Hale's parents placed calls to Cal athletic department and central administration administrators, who said they knew nothing about the incident but promised to look into it. The parents rushed by car to Alta Bates. When they arrived, after a drive of nearly two hours, no one from the university had made the comparable ten-minute drive from campus to hospital, except for one campus police officer who had been summoned to investigate. The cop said Fabiano had no recollection of how he sustained his injury, nor of anything else that day.

Eventually, the assistant coach for running backs, Pierre Ingram, arrived. Ingram told police the backstory of Hale having partied and gone out drinking on Wednesday night, causing him to miss the Thursday workout.

J.D. Hinnant, in the meantime, headed with much of the rest of the Golden Bears squad, by bus, to the Hilton Garden Inn in nearby Emeryville. Major college football teams go to the expense of putting up their players in hotels the nights before even home games. The theory is that this maximizes team bonding and minimizes distractions.

On Friday evening at the hotel, assistant coach Ingram told the campus police, according to their report, that the coaching staff intended to look into the Hinnant-Hale altercation "once [REDACTED] began to recover his memory." Ingram said he "was concerned about the players being distracted by an investigation the night before a game." The principle that a delay in interviewing third-party witnesses might degrade memories and hamper a criminal investigation evidently didn't occur to the campus cops, or at least they didn't act on any such concern.

As Hale recuperated from the assault, Hinnant was in uniform with everyone else for the Saturday game against Arizona. In the locker room, there was a rumor that the strength and conditioning staff had openly congratulated Hinnant for his forthright actions on behalf of teamwide accountability for missed conditioning drills.

When Hale recovered his memory, he seemed much less interested in pressing criminal charges than in staying in the good graces of the coaches. Two years later, the media guide biography of Harrington would include this blurb from Hale: "I've always viewed Damon as like a father figure and I've always enjoyed the relationship and his approach to life. This strength staff, they haven't just made us better on the strength side but also on the mental side, promoting and transforming us into men, where we can take on different challenges in life and maintain that same kind of focus in everything we do in life, always trying to improve ourselves and support each other to make it through."

The news media gave the incident sparse coverage. The *San Francisco Chronicle*'s Cal football beat writer reported that an unnamed "player who instigated" an intrasquad altercation of some sort was "suspended indefinitely" and required to attend counseling and perform 25 hours of community service. The newspaper also quoted a campus police lieutenant, Marc DeCoulode, as saying that "there was no evidence that hazing was involved" or that head coach Dykes "had any knowledge of this."

When I called DeCoulode myself some time later, he cut off the dialogue. "It's over and done with," the lieutenant said.

No major news outlet got around to reporting that the campus police investigation was turned over to the Alameda County district attorney's office, or that the DA spent three months coordinating a plea arrangement with Hinnant. Officially, charges against him were "deferred." In other words, the record would be expunged if Hinnant kept his nose clean through the expiration of the statute of limitations for prosecuting his offense. He did.

Players returned from the 2013–14 holiday break to a stepped-up winter conditioning program. The Golden Bears had finished Sonny Dykes's first season with a dismal record of one win and 11 losses. In the finale, Cal got humiliated by archrival Stanford, 63–13 — the most points ever scored by the winner of the "Big Game." Harrington's profane image of the Cardinal's sexual domination hit home painfully.

In his postgame news conference, and using the new coach's standard rhetorical device of blaming a bad season on the deficient talent left to him by his predecessor, Sonny Dykes said, "We're going to recruit better. We're going to recruit kids that deserve to be at Cal and want to be at Cal."

Before the student-athletes went home for the holidays, Dykes assistant Harrington circulated and made all the players sign what he labeled the "Winter Workout Contract." A facsimile of the four-page document is appended at the end of this chapter. Later, after I obtained a copy from a campus source, the university would claim to have no record of it.

The provisions of the "contract" codified a system Harrington called "the Swagger Games," whereby the team was divided into groups who competed in various benchmarks of the conditioning program. A key provision called for the group that brought up the rear in this competition, "as well as violators of the self-discipline category," to be subjected to "a massive punishment session in front of the entire team." A group finishing in last place two weeks in a row would be "required to participate in massive punishment and in addition have a workout at 5 am."

In his deposition testimony in the Agu family suit, Harrington would lie in denying the essential bullet points of the winter workout regime. The coach did acknowledge "punishment drills" in a manner he softened as "just like how I treat my kids" when they, for example, miss class, tutors, or study halls. But when asked if punishment applied when the student-athletes merely came up short in conditioning competitions, Harrington falsely answered, "No."

The pièce de résistance of the Winter Workout Contract was a drill called the "Grave digger."

On February 7, 2014, a Friday, the players were told to report to the field at Memorial Stadium, in midwinter's 6 a.m. darkness, in running sneakers rather than the shoes they used for lifting or other drills. Obviously some kind of adventure was being contemplated for outside the Simpson Center and the stadium walls. When everyone was gathered, Harrington explained a new drill he'd personally dreamed up. He called it "the Amazing Race."

Heavy, ten-foot-long cabled ropes, the kind used in tugs-of-war, were unveiled in the end zone. Groups of six players were assigned to each rope. Each group consisted of a mix of smaller backs and larger linemen, so as to keep the competition fair. The Amazing Race involved each group carrying their rope up and down a nearby campus hill ten times before finishing back inside the stadium in the end zone. The six members of each group were spaced along each rope. The ironclad rule was that everyone had to keep a grip on the rope at all times. As the saying went, "Don't let go of the rope"; everyone must support the group, which was only as strong as its weakest link. A competitive conditioning drill with a dollop of team-building.

The hill for the race led from the stadium's north tunnel entrance. Off to the right was Charter Hill, or as it's more popularly known, "Tightwad Hill," at Strawberry Canyon in the direction of the Lawrence Hall of Science much higher up. Tightwad Hill is where, during Cal football games, non-paying spectators hang out and capture freeloader views of the action inside the stadium from on high. The hill for the Amazing Race went off in a different direction, northwesterly, toward another campus landmark, the Greek Theatre. There was a path, a little more than a tenth of a mile in length, taking the players up past the parking area for a student dormitory, Bowles Hall. The slope started off gentle and got steeper.

Ted Agu, ever the leader, took up position at the front of the rope for his group, which also included Daniel Lasco. A running back, Lasco would be drafted by the NFL's New Orleans Saints in 2016 and signed to a four-year deal. (Lasco stayed with the Saints, alternating between the taxi squad and the active roster, until he suffered a spinal injury in 2017 while making a head-first tackle on a kickoff return. He was placed on injured reserve. The next year Lasco failed his preseason physical and was released.)

For the first several of the ten hill laps, the Agu group consistently led the pack or was in second place. Then Ted started laboring and fading. Lasco replaced him at the front of the rope.

Agu was not the only "big" having a hard time. In another group, a lineman complained that he couldn't feel his legs. Mindful of the team nature of the exercise, a back in that group directed the lineman to hold on to him. At one point, the big fell to the ground, rolling on the hillside several times. He was "like a boxer that had just been knocked out. You know, he was completely not there," his ropemate would testify. "Looking up, and almost crossed his eyes in the back of his head. Couldn't really tell where he was. And so we all got him up — the team. There was no effort made by anybody other than us to get him up. And we had to keep going."

Strength and conditioning coach Harrington and head athletic trainer Robbie Jackson were at the bottom of the hill in the darkness, where the road met the Bowles Hall parking lot ascent. They could observe their charges up close only once a lap. In the argot of welfare supervision, they couldn't possibly have had "eyes on" every player throughout the race.

Jackson would be the only employee of the athletic department or university management whose career was palpably harmed by that day's events. Perhaps the reason was that Agu would be the *second* sickle cell trait conditioning death on Jackson's watch. Jackson had also been a trainer at the University of Central Florida in 2008 when a player there, Ereck Plancher, died during conditioning, from what an autopsy only later unequivocally established to have been exertional sickling. (Jackson would leave the football industry and go into medical supply sales.)

On the hill, Jordan Rigsbee, an offensive guard, with blurred vision, either tripped on a pothole or simply fell. Two teammates pulled him up and he continued, walking and then jogging. When they got back to the stadium, Rigsbee profusely vomited.

Christian Okafor, another offensive lineman, fell to a knee and was in distress but kept going.

What exactly happened to Agu differed depending on whom you asked. Harrington and other team officials would testify that Agu was doing perfectly well until the very last lap, when he suffered his sole collapse. Unanimously and under oath in their own depositions, teammates said otherwise. They remembered Agu falling and struggling at least twice prior to his ultimate fatal collapse.

The objective technology of campus surveillance video was no help. In discovery, lawyers for Agu's parents would ask the university to produce video from around the stadium, but the defense lawyers told them there was no relevant video because security cameras malfunctioned.

By the players' consistent, and in my judgment more reliable, collective account, supported by detail, Agu first dropped to his knees around the sixth lap. He struggled back up. Since he was moving slower and slower, he was gradually pushed from the front of his group's rope to the back.

The second time Agu slumped over, this time with hands on knees, Lasco knew he was seriously fatigued. "Competition-wise, you never want to show your opponent you're tired or anything like that. I could tell something was definitely wrong," Lasco observed in his deposition. That was on lap seven. From there, the rest of the group told Agu to hang on while they pulled him — almost literally carried him — for two more laps.

On the tenth and final lap, with several other groups having long since passed Agu's and finished the race, Lasco and the others only wanted to be able to say that they'd completed the course. Agu sagged down for good. With words of encouragement, Lasco lifted him up under the armpits and tried to walk with him. But Agu had no legs. Near the top of the hillside, Lasco had no choice other than to ease him back to the ground. Agu told Lasco to finish with the others and leave him behind. At the same time, Lasco heard other voices shouting for trainers to rush up the hill and come to Agu's assistance.

According to witnesses, five or more minutes passed between Agu's final collapse and when head trainer Jackson and his assistant Mike Jones reached the stricken player. A golf cart was brought up, and it carried Agu back down to the north tunnel.

At 6:53 a.m., campus police officer Stephanie Martinez was in her patrol car. The radio dispatcher directed her to Memorial Stadium to assist in a medical emergency. A student-athlete "with a pre-existing medical condition" was in distress, the dispatcher said. Martinez arrived at the north tunnel at 6:57. She was carrying an automated external defibrillator device, or AED. The two athletic trainers on site were already using their own AED for cardiopulmonary resuscitation.

Language in the report later produced by another first responder, the Berkeley Fire Department's emergency medical services unit, was even more explicit than Martinez's dispatch:

ARRIVED TO FIND 20 YEAR [sic] PULSELESS AND APENIC
WITH CPR IN PROGRESS . . . PATIENT HAS HISTORY OF
SICKLE CELL [sic]

Inside the stadium, gathered near the Amazing Race's end zone finish, the players wondered if the morning's workout was over. Someone said that, following the race, the ropes might be used for tugs-of-war. But if that indeed had been the plan, it was canceled.

Addressing his troops, Harrington congratulated them for doing a good job. He also told them, "Ted is in serious trouble." Harrington said they should all say a prayer for him.

Most likely, Ted Agu was already dead.

CAL FOOTBALL
WINTER WORKOUTS – PLAYER CONTRACT

This off-season workout is designed to help each individual player reach their maximum potential both in the weight room and on the field by becoming bigger, faster and stronger. Our team goal is to win a pac-12 championship and this can only be achieved through sacrifice, discipline and dedication. This means that despite ANY circumstances that come, you place the team above self and all work toward a common goal. We will win our games this fall by how we work starting in January. **Earn the right to be successful!**

1. I WILL ALWAYS BE ON TIME! 1 SECOND LATE IS LATE.
2. IF I HAVE A CONFLICT, I WILL COMMUNICATE WITH STRENGTH COACHES AND HAVE A <u>VALID</u> REASON B/F MY SCHEDULED LIFT/RUN. FAILURE TO COMMUNICATE WILL BE CONSIDERED AN ABSENCE.
   DAMON- ▓▓▓▓▓▓
   SAL- ▓▓▓▓▓▓
   MAHALA- ▓▓▓▓▓▓
3. IF I'M SICK, I WILL PHYSICALLY REPORT TO THE TRAINING ROOM B/F MY SCHEDULED LIFT/RUN TO BE EXCUSED. CALLING FROM BED IS NOT CONSIDERED EXCUSED.
4. I WILL BE COACHABLE AND TAKE CONSTRUCTIVE CRITICISM.
5. ONLY CAL ISSUED APPAREL WILL BE WORN. THIS INCLUDES NO EAR RINGS, NECKLACES, SOCKS, HEADGEAR, ETC. THERE WILL BE NO MODIFICATION TO ISSUED GEAR. I AM WILLING TO SACRIFICE MY INDIVIDUALITY TO CONEORM INTO ONE COHESIVE TEAM.
6. I WILL NEVER MAKE EXCUSES FOR MYSELF OR MY TEAMMATES. I WILL OWN MY ACTIONS.
7. I WILL GIVE MY ALL FOR MY TEAMMATES AND **ABOVE ALL ELSE FOR CAL** AND OUR SUCCESS ON A DAILY BASIS.
8. I WILL BE GRATEFUL FOR THIS OPPORTUNITY AND AS SUCH, WILL NOT ACT ENTITLED OR COMPLAIN AS I UNDERSTAND THAT I CHOSE TO BE A PART OF THIS TEAM.

IF I VIOLATE ANY OF THESE RULES, I WILL BE HELD ACCOUNTABLE BY BOTH TEAMMATES AND COACHES AND SUBJECT TO ANY DISCIPLINE AS A RESULT OF MY ACTIONS.

- Team will be divided into 8 teams
- Each team will have a captain chosen by the coaching staff
- Captains will name teams
- Draft will be held by captains before competition start
- Coaches will be drafted to teams
- Draft will be posted so each person on our team knows where they stand with their teammates

Draft:
1. Draft order will be determined by drawing numbers from a hat
2. Order will go 1-8/8-1 for each round. Each round will have specific picks as follows:
   Rd 1 – wildcard
   Rd 2 – OL/DL
   Rd 3 – LB/TE/SP/FB
   Rd 4 – WR/DB/RB/QB
   <Repeat Order Rds 5-8>

Competition points will be drawn from 6 categories. Those categories are as follows:

1. Speed
2. Agilities
3. Strength
4. Academics
5. Self-Discipline
6. Combative

1. SPEED (M/TH)

- Groups will be divided by speed level with up to 8 groups from fastest to slowest
- Will run 6-8 sprints up to 25-30 yds or until required yardage of 250 yds
- Every race will have a winner and a loser who will be awarded points
- Winner (+1)
- Loser (-1)
- Points will be totaled at end of running session and awarded to overall team points
- Winners with most points totaled will adjust up a group to a faster speed level
- Losers with most negative points totaled will adjust down to a slower speed level

Competitions: Monday - Race (3 pt)   Thursday - Tires
                Reaction   Hills
                2 pt   Steps
                Seated
                200's
                400's
                COD Sprints

Manpower: Starter
                Winner
                Loser
                2 scribes

2. **AGILITIES (TU/FRI)**

   Phase I — weight staff
   - 4 stations per half/ 8 total (2 teams per station)
   - 1 vs. 1 every drill/play on each team
   - Winner awarded +1
   - Loser awarded -1

   Examples of Drills:

   1. Pro agility
   2. L-Drill
   3. 60 yd shuttle
   4. 3 bag drill
   5. 4 cone drills
   6. Hoop drill
   7. 6 bag drill
   8. 6 cone drill
   9. 40 yd shuttle

   Phase II(coaches) - mat agilities

   Examples of Drills:

   1. Quarter eagles
   2. Shuffle wave + up down
   3. 2 pt seat roll
   4. 4 pt seat roll
   5. 4-way run
   6. 2-way run/shuffle
   7. 4 pt bear and roll

   Manpower: Coach and scribe with each team

   - Coach and scribe will rotate with teams each station
   - Points can/will be calculated at half time and after agilities are completed
   - Coaches have option to condition entire team at half time
   - Losing 4 teams will also condition after agilities are completed

3. **ACADEMICS**

   - Points will be (+) or (-) per Academic team

     (+) points – attendance
     　　　　　　Work ethic
     　　　　　　Attitude
     　　　　　　Grades

     (-) points – study hall
     　　　　　　class
     　　　　　　tutors
     　　　　　　attitude
     　　　　　　Grades

4. **SELF DISCIPLINE**

   (+) points – Exceptional attitude
   　　　　　　Discipline
   　　　　　　Team member
   　　　　　　Effort/work ethic
   　　　　　　Toughness
   　　　　　　Bodyweight
   　　　　　　Body Language

   (-) points – Missed/late workout
   　　　　　　Missed/late treatment
   　　　　　　Attitude
   　　　　　　Effort/work ethic
   　　　　　　Toughness
   　　　　　　Bodyweight
   　　　　　　Body Language

5. STRENGTH

- Will be done in or after workout
- All competitions will be timed
- Record results all day and take average of team or total number of reps per team
- First place team will receive 8 pts with rest according to where team finishes down to 1 pt

  Examples of competitions: Push ups
  Pull ups
  Bench press
  Dips
  Plate holds
  Sit ups
  Bar Hangs

- Strength coaches reserve the right to award points for outstanding feats of strength, such as PR's, etc.

6. COMBATIVE

Phase I – 10 combats a day
Phase II – incorporate into agilities

Examples of combative drills:

1. Thunderdome *
2. Death Crawl *
3. Tug of War*
4. Terrible Towel*
5. Tire of Terror
6. Tire Tap Out
7. Grave digger

*incorporate into sand pit
- Combative drills can be scheduled into workouts or at end of run or done at any point during those things with the element of surprise

NOTES:

- Points will be calculated throughout week
- At the end of every week, points will be posted
- A massive punishment session in front of the entire team featuring the previous weeks losing team as well as violators of self-discipline category. All players/coaches are required to attend.
- Winning team will be rewarded from previous week at punishment session.
- If a team is in last place 2 week in a row, they will be required to participate in massive punishment and in addition have a workout at 5 am.

CHAPTER 3

Anatomy
of a
Cover-Up

C over-ups are not all-or-nothing affairs; they occur on a continuum. In the case of Cal-Berkeley's Ted Agu death clean-up operation — a textbook execution of corporate reputational hygiene — it aligned conveniently with its intended audience's biases. This helped make it more palatable. For sure, it wasn't as extreme as something like the My Lai massacre. It was more like the ongoing fudging of Vietnam War casualty statistics by Robert McNamara's generals.

Still, its essence was clear. Ted Agu died of exertional sickling. The university and its football program were content to have the public cling, either permanently or at least for as long as possible, to the fiction that Agu was felled by a heart attack. In one quick-hit local newspaper account the next day, the player was said to have collapsed while jogging on campus with his buddies.

The cover-up would get exposed in a limited way by the Agu family's lawsuit against the University of California Regents, which settled in 2016 for $4.75 million. But survivors' monetary recoveries — the only kind of restitution the system seems to know how to fashion out of their horrible losses — aren't the equivalent of fulfillment of the public interest in fully appreciating what happened and why.

More comprehensively, the university's cover-up would be exposed by the output of my California Public Records Act petition against the university, filed in state court in 2017. More than 700 pages of previously withheld documents, some of them critical to the narrative of actions taken to deflect attention from the university's negligence in managing Agu's susceptibility to exertional sickling, were released over the course of several years, in the wake of court orders.

In 2021, a judge in the Superior Court of Alameda County ruled that I was the prevailing party for having "catalyzed" these productions, and that my attorney, Roy S. Gordet, was entitled to reimbursement of attorney fees. The judge directed the parties to negotiate Gordet's fees, and they submitted to the court the terms of a settlement for $125,000, which got incorporated into the court's final judgment.

The university then appealed the whole thing to California's First District Court of Appeal. The Reporters Committee for Freedom of the Press and the California First Amendment Coalition filed an amicus curiae, or "friend of the court," brief on my behalf. UC, the amici wrote, seek "to chill future litigation by public records requesters and deter investigative reporting." But the appellate panel, reversing the lower court, held that the university, not I, was the prevailing party. The production of new public records related to the management of the Agu death, the appellate justices said, had not, after all, been "catalyzed" by my taking the institution to court and by my lawyer's years of litigating the Public Records Act petition. Rather, the new documents were merely the result of the university's own extra efforts, at the prodding of the trial court.

This amounted to theorizing that the significant new public information pointing to a cover-up had spontaneously combusted, or perhaps been produced out of the goodness of the hearts of the practitioners of the cover-up.

At Superior Court, the UC Regents had further moved for the judge to find that my Public Records Act petition was "clearly frivolous," kicking in monetary sanctions to punish me for my supposedly unprecedented squandering of judicial resources over a matter of such hilarity and to deter future such jesters. After losing that motion in lower court, the university doubled down on it on appeal. Like the Superior Court, the Court of Appeal refused to go that far. I speculate that the appellate justices might have viewed the simultaneous cancellation of reimbursement of my own legal fees as some exquisitely Solomonic compromise.

All this, of course, was long removed from the contemporaneous headlines of Ted Agu's death. By the time of the appellate fight — a series of events as ignored by major news media as were the circumstances of the original fatality giving rise to it — any competent damage control consultant would have counseled UC that, by blurring the public's immediate grasp of the events reported in the previous chapter, the university had already spectacularly triumphed. By 2022, a finding of who was on the hook for the records act requester's legal fees was almost extraneous. And for the multibillion-dollar university, the disputed $125,000 in fees that it was ordered to pay, prior to the appellate court reversal, was taxicab money.

Ultimately, the proof is in the pudding of the information footprint. From the initial months through as much as four and a half years later, anyone doing basic research on the Internet's Google search engine would see on a search for "Ted Agu cause of death" the top-line result "hypertrophic cardiomyopathy" or HCM: thickening of the heart muscle. Only very recently did this Google result fall away — replaced by links to various news articles in 2016 more accurately recording that while the Alameda County medical examiner's first autopsy finding was HCM, that office later revised its report to acknowledge exertional sickling as a "contributing" factor.

In fact, a heart condition "contributed" to Ted Agu's exertional sickling death approximately the same way a stoppage of breathing "contributes" to the deaths of schoolchildren in gun massacres. The University of California's ability to stonewall, then slow-walk, an accurate official cause of death finding affirmed the old quip, often attributed to Mark Twain, about how a lie gets halfway around the world before the truth puts its boots on. Today few remember or care who Ted Agu was, or that he died. Or that there was ever a dispute over how he died. Or that any of it matters.

Recording the opposite here is one small way to register that if the band doesn't fail to play on, then at least it can be compelled to take a musicians-union-mandated break.

The cover-up quarterback for Cal was Dr. Casey Batten, the football team physician. First, do no harm — to football world.

The record shows that in the immediate hours or days following Agu's death — the established timeline isn't exact — Batten placed an unsolicited phone call to the chief forensics officer, Dr. Thomas Beaver. Their conversation had the effect of putting a thumb on the scale of the investigation by Beaver and the office supervising him, the Alameda County sheriff. From the known facts of what Batten did, blurring the efforts of an investigation by a police agency, an aggressive prosecutor would have all the evidence needed, in his or her discretion, to indict for obstruction of justice. This was close to the sports equivalent of President Donald Trump's call to the Georgia secretary of state asking him to find extra votes to flip the state's Electoral College victory from Joe Biden.

Without qualification, Batten asserted to Beaver that, in his considered professional opinion as the medical authority at closest proximity at the time of the incident, Agu's death appeared to be an open-and-shut case of HCM. Batten didn't seem to deem it worth mentioning that Agu was a known sickle cell trait carrier, even though the near-certainty that he'd succumbed in a sickling episode was dominating internal university discussion at the very moment he placed the call. In fact, Batten never even got around to uttering the words "sickle cell."

For the part of the medical examiner — judging from his own later deposition testimony — it's questionable whether Dr. Beaver had ever even heard of the syndrome of exertional sickling before holding that the cause of death was HCM.

As noted earlier, head football coach Sonny Dykes emerged just fine from presiding over a program in which a student-athlete died from gross negligence, if not outright criminality. Eventually Dykes did get fired at Berkeley, but that was only because of a losing record and declining attendance, combined with the administration's pique over his ongoing undisguised courtship of other jobs. A drop in season ticket numbers was especially worrisome, since the university was managing (and continues to face) many tens of millions of dollars of debt service in the earthquake retrofitting and upgrade of Memorial Stadium. This has forced massive diversions of funds from academic programs to offset athletic department budget deficits.

The death of a student-athlete on Dykes's watch had nothing to do with why he had to go. Subsequent to the university's multimillion-dollar settlement with the Agu family, Dykes had even leveraged that contract extension and raise. Cal was just a career stepping stone. And today he's the hottest name in college football coaching.

When Dykes departed Cal, so did Damon Harrington, his strength and conditioning assistant. In a perverse twist, the coach whose excesses spurred the demise of a carrier of sickle cell trait moved to Grambling State University in Louisiana, a prominent historically Black school. (In 2020, Harrington left Grambling for the same position at Texas State.)

Sandy Barbour, Cal's athletic director when Agu died, migrated to AD at Penn State later in 2014. She retired in 2022.

Dr. Casey Batten's career turned out just fine too. In 2016, he became lead primary care physician for the NFL's Los Angeles Rams. In fairness to Batten, it must be added that at Berkeley, he was merely loyally following the directions, or at least the perceived wishes, of the athletic department and the central administration officials to whom he reported.

In further fairness, let's note that Batten (who never responded to my multiple inquiries) did testify under oath about his meddling phone call to the medical examiner prior to the cutting of Agu's corpse. Unfortunately, Batten's account fell a bit short in the coherence department. According to the court reporter's transcript, he stammered:

> Umm, I don't recall that I had a conversation where we — I think
> we did say something along the lines of [Agu's death] appeared to
> be, but it was — I think it was — it might have been after — I really
> don't recall when I spoke with him.

Cal scheduled an afternoon news conference to discuss the tragedy at the morning football practice. At 12:55 p.m., around six hours after Agu was pronounced dead, Wesley Mallette of the athletic department's sports information office circulated by email, to Dr. Batten and others who'd be taking the podium in front of live local cable TV cameras, a script of questions and answers. The very first anticipated question was: "Was there anything in Ted's medical background that would lead you to believe something like this could happen?"

Batten was coached to reply — and at the media briefing did reply — "At this time, we are precluded by law to comment on any other medical details and out of respect for the family and the situation." (One of the laws purportedly at play was an excessively cited and utterly irrelevant federal statute, the Family Educational Rights and Privacy Act, or FERPA. More later on the university's abuse of FERPA as a cover-up crutch. The privacy rules of HIPAA, the Health Insurance Portability and Accountability Act, also had dubious application to the circumstances of the death in the course of a publicly commercial activity.)

In answer to questions about the events of early morning, the doctor said that toward the end of the workout the staff noticed that Ted was having difficulty. "As a precaution, his activity was immediately stopped and he was attended to." Further, and again "as a precaution," he was placed on a cart and taken 150 yards toward the medical facility in the stadium "for observation and treatment." Agu was alert and responsive until they reached the north tunnel — at which point he no longer was. CPR was administered and EMS was summoned.

Perhaps inadvertently, Batten's own canned account, even in this inaccurate form (A single collapse? Necessitating measures "as a precaution"?), was perfectly consistent with a diagnosis of ES and perfectly inconsistent with one of HCM. In ES, medical experts say, the muscles give out first as the heart still beats strong. When an athlete in these straits goes to the ground, he typically can still talk and follow commands. Over the next up to 20 minutes, though, his condition deteriorates in the midst of a "metabolic storm" brought on by the explosive muscle breakdown caused by rhabdomyolysis. Dead muscle tissue enters the bloodstream. Only at that point does even a normal heart stop. This differs from an HCM episode, in which the heart was structurally abnormal and the collapse was caused by a dire cardiac arrhythmia. In that circumstance, such a victim would probably hit the ground hard, say nothing, and be unconscious within seconds. Unless the heart quickly got shocked back into normal rhythm, he would be dead almost instantaneously; he would not deteriorate in stages.

Either just before or, more likely, a short time after, Batten no-commented to reporters on grounds of the "privacy" of a dead person, Batten placed his autopsy-investigation-obstructing phone call to Beaver. The forensic pathologist would cut and examine Agu's body three days later.

Cal officials did some decent, basic, expected things for the Agu family. That is to say, they supported the funeral in Bakersfield. They staged a candlelight vigil on campus and moments of silence before upcoming intercollegiate sports events, the first of which was a women's volleyball match. And they started making arrangements for the Memorial Stadium plaque honoring Ted.

Parallel with all that, they carried out a PR plumbing operation.

Teresa Kuehn Gould, a deputy to athletic director Barbour, emailed seven department officials that she was gathering "some of the basic questions we anticipate our staff getting." The first of the eight questions was even more explicit than the sports information office's had been for Batten and the others at the same-day press conference: "Did Ted test positive for sickle cell trait?" The evasive answer, with the privacy-respecting excuse, remained the same.

The second question was, "How can we prevent this from happening again?" Gould's first draft of the frequently asked questions document suggested the answer: "Right now, we don't know why Ted passed away and we are working to find those answers. But as with any instance when you experience a tragedy such as this, it gives cause to go back and look over your protocols and procedures to make sure you are doing everything possible should you be faced with a worse case [sic] scenario situation."

That answer was way too forthcoming for Ryan Cobb, the associate athletic director for performance, health, and welfare. In a group email conference, he walked it back to: "We will continue to operate within all NCAA and medical best practices, and hope to have answers specific to Ted as they become available to us."

Another deputy athletic director, Phil Esten, was the official who stayed on top of references in social media and on the discussion boards of legacy media websites. As reported to his colleagues, Esten was especially concerned with an anonymous poster at sfgate.com, then the site of *San Francisco Chronicle* content. Among other alarming statements, that person claimed to have "witnesses" who saw Dr. Batten, head coach Dykes, and athletic director Barbour "huddled up" outside Alta Bates hospital, where Agu had been rushed, "to decide how to cover their asses," as the poster put it.

A Cal Sports marketing employee, Andy Lempart, told Esten, "The person seems to have some sort of access based on their comments."

Barbour herself didn't think anyone saw her with others at Alta Bates. However, she admitted in an email, "It's certainly possible" that outsiders might have gotten inside another crisis precinct, the football facility, in the midst of the chaos that day.

Asten told the email discussion thread, "It looks like most comments are positive. There were a few sickle cell comments on Bear Insider and Jim McGill [editor-in-chief of this athletic department news website] asked that people don't speculate."

As university image–minders braced for withering criticism, they got a gift in the form of public remarks by Bret Bielema, the head football coach at Arkansas. Bielema was in the midst of campaigning for rules changes to curtail "hurry up" offenses, in which the pace of play is picked up by abandoning the huddle, as a way to keep the defense off balance. Sonny Dykes's Air Raid system was one of several offensive schemes that often go no-huddle. In an online interview with *Sports Illustrated*, Bielema implied that hurry-ups heightened pressure for cardiovascular conditioning rigor, which in turn endangered lives. Asked for evidence that hurry-ups translated to such risks, Bielema pointed to what he called a clear answer: "Death certificates. There's no more anything I need than that." Bielema also noted that Agu had sickle cell trait — something Cal wasn't yet acknowledging.

Bielema got almost universally panned for speculating about a cause of death that wasn't established. Even worse than the substance was the style: Bielema's tastelessness in injecting the Agu tragedy into a debate over in-game competition rules.

In Berkeley, decision-makers mulled their most effective moral-high-ground ripostes. The sports information office's Mallette coordinated consideration of a "strategic approach" for registering their outrage over the exploitation of their tragedy by an outsider coach in service of his own campaign for rules changes. At the conclusion of Agu's funeral in Bakersfield, Sandy Barbour settled on issuing a series of four posts on Twitter:

> 1. Today our @CalFootball #CalFamily lays to rest one of our own. Ted Agu — forever in our hearts.
>
> 2. Thanks to all for the tremendous support with the loss of Ted Agu. Means the world to Ted's and our #CalFamily.
>
> 3. Bret Bielema's comments about our Ted Agu are misinformed, ill-advised and beyond insensitive.
>
> 4. Using the tragic loss of one of our student-athletes as a platform to further a personal agenda in a public setting is repulsive.

In the ensuing Twitter backlash, Bielema apologized for inflicting "unintended hurt." Even if it was only momentary, the Cal Sports and university administrators were relieved to be leaning into some PR offense on the Ted Agu story.

Bielema "is being crushed in the media," Mallette enthused in an email to Barbour. "Your Tweets went over well and NBCSports.com positioned us appropriately."

At 9:30 a.m. on February 11, four days after Agu's death, Damon Harrington was summoned to the campus police station for an interview. According to the transcript, Detective Harry Bennigson told the strength and conditioning coach that "Decco" — Lieutenant Marc DeCoulode — "has asked me to look into this" and to make sure "there's nothing suspicious about it."

"There's rumors about sickle cell anemia [*sic*]," Bennigson said.

In a preamble, the detective attempted to bond with Harrington by bragging about his own football background, rambling about the challenges of conditioning, and reassuring the coach that the Cal program was not under scrutiny. He himself had "played a little college ball uh, back in my days, the '70s," at a junior college, Bennigson said. In those days, "we took salt tablets. . . . I don't think you've ever heard that, but [that was] all we knew back then." His college line coach "was big on the hills. Oh my God, he would make us run up and walk down."

Coming off like a bumpkin, Bennigson continued on the theme of exuding sympathy for the interviewee. In interview technique, such a ploy can be designed to wheedle cooperation and information, but no such agenda seemed in play here. Instead, the campus police were just underscoring for an employee of the football program that they were all in this together.

Bennigson soliloquized that a football team is "just a tight group" and "law enforcement's the same way. . . . I don't think, unless you're involved in that, nobody knows the tightness, you know. It's almost like being a Marine or something."

The detective said, "I hate to see a death, but this is going to bring everybody closer. . . . I mean, this is going to make them probably play even tougher, you know, cause they're going to want to play for him." He even called the tragic scenario "neat," in the limited sense that "it does bring people tighter together."

"By no means," Bennigson told Harrington, "are we trying to put a blame on anything. . . . We're not looking into what conditioning program is or nothing like that. That's . . . uh, some people are asking, 'Well, what are you guys — are you going to be looking into the program?' 'No.'" He added: "I mean, to me, it looks like it's going to be some kind of a natural cause. So uh, you know. It's just unfortunate and it happens."

Bennigson moved on to a handful of softball questions about the previous Friday.

This "interrogation," however, must not have been good enough for Lieutenant DeCoulode, who called Harrington back to the police station an hour later for a do-over. During this second interview, DeCoulode sat in and sometimes added his own questions to those of Bennigson. According to the supplemental report, the purpose of the follow-up "was to clarify information regarding AGU's medical condition":

> Lt. DeCoulode asked HARRINGTON a hypothetical question. "In your medical training, if someone had a medical condition Sickle Cell Trait, are there any specific things that you should watch for or do differently?"
>
> HARRINGTON replied by saying that he worked with a number of those types of athletes before. Not necessarily at UC Berkeley, but at other colleges. HARRINGTON explained that he "would look for cramping and other signs of difficulty [such as] breathing problems."

When Bennigson asked him about sickle cell trait in the second interview, Harrington expressed uncertainty over whether he could disclose private medical information. Bennigson said, "Well, I think because it's an investigation you can." Under DeCoulode's prodding, Bennigson stepped up his game one more notch, to flat-out witness-coaching:

> Q   So w- if you're not comfortable answering that . . .
>
> A   Mm-hm.
>
> Q   . . . you can say that you were aware that he had medical conditions but you don't wanna say specifically what they were.
>
> A   Okay.
>
> Q   But my understanding earlier was that when you were asked if you knew of any medical conditions . . .
>
> A   Mm-hm.
>
> Q   . . . you said no or you weren't very specific.
>
> A   I said I don't know.
>
> Q   Right.

A   I — I mean, like . . .

Q   S- so keep in mind what we don't wanna do is we don't wanna
have it appear that you're either not telling the truth . . .

A   Mm-hm.

Q   . . . or that you're being deceptive.

Harrington opened up enough to allow that if any players "have a medical condition we are informed because, I mean, we have to know . . ." Beyond that, "I'd rather not elaborate."

Two weeks later, Detective Bennigson interviewed Mike Jones, the assistant athletic trainer. Bennigson recorded: "I asked JONES if he was aware of any medical condition with AGU. JONES told me that he knew of AGU's medical status but he did not know if he was allowed to talk about it."

A number of Agu's teammates were distraught and felt the true story was getting buried. A quarterback deep in the roster depth chart, Joey Mahalic, was more than distraught; he was, if not enraged, then certainly confused.

Mahalic was part of the non-travel group who'd been subjected to Harrington's Thursday punishment drills. In that capacity, Mahalic had witnessed the Fabiano Hale–J.D. Hinnant incident the previous November. In addition, Mahalic had participated in the "Amazing Race" drill that killed Agu. Mahalic connected these events as elements of a toxic program that needed to be addressed and corrected. But he didn't know quite how to go about it.

Mahalic's first sport had been baseball: he was drafted by the Cleveland Indians (now Guardians) as a pitcher out of Wilson High School in Portland, Oregon, before injuring his arm and getting released. His father, Drew Mahalic, after playing linebacker at Notre Dame and for four years in the NFL, had become a lawyer, earning his degree from Harvard. Joey consulted with his dad.

Joey also had a friend in some of his classes who had been a colonel in the Marines, and after his service hitch, pursued higher education studies.

The friend advised him to take his concerns to university officials. Mahalic spoke with Solly Fulp, a deputy athletic director; athletic director Sandy Barbour; physics professor Bob Jacobsen, the faculty athletics adviser; and John Wilton, the university's vice chancellor for finance and administration. Wilton promised Mahalic there would be a "third-party investigation." Jacobsen steered him to the campus police.

On March 19, Detective Bennigson interviewed Mahalic. The student-athlete told the whole Hinnant-Hale story and laid out "the culture that the strength coach is trying to set up. Um, you know, if you're working out and you're throwing up, you have to keep going through the drill and still be throwing up. You can't be bending down to throw up or anything like that. Um, so that's kind of the mentality that we have. So take that coming into Friday [the day of Agu's death]."

Mahalic reiterated that his concerns went all the way back to November, "after the Fabiano [Hale] thing, where I said, 'I probably need to say something right now.'" Mahalic didn't interpret the incident as the fault of either Hale or J.D. Hinnant, but rather "being bullied by a strength guy."

Bennigson thanked Mahalic for his time.

In March, Vice Chancellor Wilton emailed the campus police chief, Margo Bennett. "When we talked recently about the Agu incident," Wilton said, "you said you would pull all the work your dept. has done together and send it to me. How is that coming along?"

Bennett obliged by giving the vice chancellor copies of a batch of documents. "I am fairly confident that Sandy [athletic director Barbour] has not had access to this level of detail," the police chief confided. In any case, "please don't share the papers . . . I put them together for you (and [Wilton's assistant] Ann if needed) only. If others need the information, I am happy to give a verbal briefing, but not documents. The case is not available for a PRA [Public Records Act] request and I'd like to keep it that way."

Ever since Dr. Batten had worked the referee in the autopsy investigation with his irregular call to the forensic pathologist, locking him onto hypertrophic cardiomyopathy as the cause of Agu's death while scrupulously avoiding any reference to exertional sickling, Cal officials were sweating out the release of the medical examiner's report. Everyone was pretty sure Dr. Beaver had little or no inkling of sickle cell trait and its implications. Still, a cover-up is never over until it's over.

Lieutenant DeCoulode used his contacts in the county sheriff's office to play point through this vigil. On April 21, he sent an email with what his audience would receive as emphatically good news. The email went to Chief Bennett, athletic director Barbour, chief campus lawyer Christopher Patti, chief campus media spokesperson Dan Mogulof, and athletic department PR executive Herb Benenson.

"This morning I was informed by the Coroner's office that the cause of death for Ted Agu is natural, due to Hypertrophic cardiomyopathy," DeCoulode wrote. "Below is a brief description of Hypertrophic cardiomyopathy from the internet. The Coroner's office will likely release this to the media this afternoon."

The report included the coroner office's Beaver's rundown from when he cut into Agu's corpse in February. He didn't say so, but of course this was shortly after team physician Batten's call pushing the theory of HCM. Beaver did note that "some of the red blood cells within some of the blood vessels have morphology consistent with 'sickle cell disease.' However, this could be the result of low oxygen tension either antemortem or postmortem."

So it would indeed go down as HCM. Not ES. That was the official finding. But it wouldn't be the last word.

Though Detective Bennigson had assured Damon Harrington that his strength and conditioning program was not being investigated, the university did seem to realize that someone, one or more independent experts, needed to be enlisted at least to go through the motions of doing some sort of probe confirming everything was on the up-and-up. And Wilton had given Mahalic assurances of something to that effect.

Performance chief Ryan Cobb became the athletic department official tasked with helping commission what he called, in an email to Barbour, a "'review.'" (The ironic or scare quotes were Cobb's own.) To co-author the study, Cobb selected Dr. Jeffrey Tanji, a sports medicine specialist at UC Davis, and John Murray, a freelance athletic trainer in San Francisco.

To call the independence of the "review" questionable would be an understatement. Tanji met with Dr. Batten at a medical convention in New Orleans just a week before starting on his work on the conditioning program report. And he and Murray both had ties to Cal Sports. Nonetheless, on March 31 the campus counsel, Patti, drafted a letter for Vice Chancellor Wilton with the terms of the Tanji-Murray review and its charging instructions.

The next day, Tanji told Cobb that he proposed "to interview appropriate members of the students, coaches, ATCs, and team physicians during a one day period of time. . . . [I want] to be very respectful of all of our time and handle this in the most efficient way possible."

Usually, investigators ask questions until there are no longer any nontrivial open ones. But this particular investigator tailored his work to the convenience of the subjects of his investigation. The phrase "once over lightly" is too kind.

Cobb put together an itinerary for Tanji in Berkeley and worked on the logistics of booking an interview room at the Simpson Center, as well as "refining the list of who will be interviewed, with those you have identified and filling the others in consult with Sandy [athletic director Barbour], UC Administration."

An independent investigation for which the lead investigator doesn't at the very least decide, in his sole discretion, whom to interview or attempt to interview?

Tanji told Cobb he was declining a per diem payment. Tanji called the job a "professional courtesy for my colleagues." Tanji had a concept, however, for where the university might put up both his wife and himself for one day. His wife "already has a place in mind," Tanji said. That place was the posh Claremont Club & Spa in the hills on the Berkeley-Oakland border.

On April 9, Cobb updated his boss, Barbour, on the status of the "review." Dr. Tanji was set to visit the campus later in the month, and Fulp, the deputy AD, would "think further about which football players to include." Cobb calculated that it would be sufficient to interview from three to eight football players. But on April 15, citing "a push from Athletics to include more student-athletes," Cobb suggested to Tanji that they upgrade to "you seeing 8 of them, 20 minutes each, for a total of 16 over 4 total hours." (In addition, Coach Dykes had insisted on talking to the full team about the review before the interviews took place, and on meeting himself with Tanji and Murray.)

"We just want to make sure we include you in all these decisions," Cobb told Tanji — again turning on its head every standard of best practices in an independent investigation.

Tanji and Murray wound up talking to a total of 15 players, according to a spreadsheet later leaked to me by a campus source (yet never produced by the university in response to Public Records Act requests). Fourteen others were contacted, but either declined to be interviewed or didn't respond to an invitation. Sources said the names were generated by a random computer algorithm working from the full roster of student-athletes. J.D. Hinnant, the player who'd criminally assaulted and battered Fabiano Hale, was one of those contacted. My information doesn't make clear whether Hale was contacted. It's believed that Joey Mahalic, whose whistle-blower actions all the way through the interview with the campus police had helped necessitate the review, was *not* part of the Tanji interview group, for whatever reason.

On May 23, Tanji gave Cobb a progress report. "I will have this done in less than a week. In summary, it will be a positive report," Tanji promised.

Not only positive — also extremely short. On June 9, Tanji submitted a document to Wilton that barely ran onto a fourth page, one-and-a-half-spaced (including final paragraphs simply disclosing the authors' relationships with the athletic department). Relevant excerpts:

The Four Questions

1. Are the program's training practices, and in particular, the intensity of workouts, consistent with protection of student-athlete health and safety with training practices in college and university sports programs at this level?

[Yes.]

. . .

2. Has the strength and conditioning staff used training inappropriately for punitive purposes?

No, they have not used training inappropriately. It is not
unusual to have a team do additional drills for a missed practice, but this was not done inappropriately in our review.

During the interview process an incident came to light
raised by one of the members of the athletic training staff.
During the season one member of the football team punched
another member of the team in the locker room for not
participating in a workout which resulted in the team having
to do additional training. While the athlete who punched
was suspended — the sentiment was that this athlete "sent a
message from the rest of the team" to the athlete who missed
the workout. The other athletes not directly involved in the
incident felt that this was not encouraged or sanctioned by
the strength and conditioning staff, but the action of one
athlete to another.

. . .

3. Have strength and conditioning coaches used abusive language
or engaged in abusive action toward players?

. . . [N]o one interviewed felt that [profanity] was focused on
an athlete in an abusive fashion, or at the team in an abusive
manner.

. . .

4. Is the level of medical monitoring of workouts appropriate and has the medical team responded appropriately when student-athletes have shown signs of distress?

   The level of medical monitoring and awareness of student-athlete pre-existing conditions, current injuries and distress are appropriate both in a general sense and in the specific case of Ted Agu, the student-athlete who met an untimely death in February 2014.

Meanwhile, the Agu family lawsuit wended its way through the Alameda County Superior Court docket. In depositions, several players corroborated Mahalic's account of Harrington's excesses, including his at least indirect incitement of Hinnant's attack on Hale.

Riddic Bowers, an Alameda County sheriff's lieutenant, was shown campus police reports totaling 141 pages that had been produced in discovery. The last chapter of this batch consisted of the dozen or so pages from his own office, in April and June 2014, closing the medical examiner's autopsy report. But unquestionably, there was also a collection of campus police records, contemporaneous with the Agu death investigation, totaling well over 100 other pages. These included the interview of Mahalic and the two interviews of Harrington — Detective Bennigson's original plus the Lieutenant DeCoulode–assisted do-over. Bowers testified that Cal had faxed only 29 total pages to the sheriff. What happened to these and other reports?

Chief forensic pathologist Beaver (who by then had left Alameda County for the same job at a municipality in Florida) was confronted with all this information and asked about Batten's call to him and other discrepancies:

A [D]id Dr. Batten ever tell you that Ted Agu had sickle cell trait?

Q No, he did not.

A Okay. So sickle cell trait was not even in your mind at the time you talked to Dr. Batten the day of your autopsy and your cutting young Agu?

Q   That's correct. [. . .] [I]t didn't even cross my mind.

A   Okay. And having been told that Ted Agu collapsed suddenly, did you then begin to initially believe or lead you to believe that there may be a cardiac death?

Q   Yes.

A   Okay. If you'd been told that Ted Agu struggled over a period of many minutes, gradually got worse, did not collapse suddenly, may have collapsed several times until the ultimate collapse, would sickle cell trait have been a consideration at that time?

. . .

A   [M]y interpretation of [others'] deposition testimony is that Ted Agu was ill for a period of time [. . .]

. . .

[W]hat I could see from reading the depositions of different players that were in the drill with him is — and they varied, as you said. There was, there was various laps and various times and, and so it, it wasn't consistent, but, but the one thing that was consistent is that there was this period of time. It wasn't a sudden collapse. It wasn't as if he took a knee and died. That, and that was what I was looking at initially. So there's this period of being, being ill, being sick, being tired, being, you know, decompensating, so he had this period of decompensation prior to his cardiac arrest. So in that, in that context that's, that is more consistent with a, a death from, from a sickle crisis than it is a death from a sudden cardiac dysrhythmia from hypertrophic myocardiopathy in my opinion.

. . .

So in my opinion based upon all of the information that I have today as we sit here is that the cause of death is best certified as sickle cell crisis or complications of sickle cell crisis and, and I think that is, outweighs the hypertrophic cardiomyopathy.

In 2021, Beaver (by then on the faculty of the Medical University of South Carolina) put it to me this way: "I was fully aware of exertional sickling when I did the autopsy, but I had no history of sickle cell disease or trait." In examining Agu's body, he found "mild to moderate cardiomegaly" (an enlarged heart) but no evidence of HCM or hypertensive cardiovascular disease. "I was given the history that he was perfectly healthy and had participated in this specific drill many times without the slightest issue. It was not until I looked at the cardiac biopsy material that I found sickle cell in the microvasculature and could raise the issue." From that point forward, Beaver said, the investigation was conducted by the sheriff's office and he was no longer involved. "I was never given the history of documented sickle cell trait, or shown any documentation that I recall."

Following his deposition, Beaver took the extraordinary step of writing to his old colleagues at the Alameda County sheriff's office and requesting a change in the original finding of the cause of Ted Agu's death. According to the revised finding, exertional sickling was upgraded from no mention to a contributory cause. A facsimile of the Beaver letter is appended to the end of this chapter.

Talks between the University of California's lawyers and the Agu family's intensified to hammer out their lawsuit settlement.

When Rashidi Wheeler perished at Northwestern in 2001, scrutiny of the incident by Chicago's major daily newspapers, the *Tribune* and the *Sun-Times*, was relentless. The infamous video described in Chapter 1 — provided to the media by family lawyer Johnnie Cochran — got broken down and commented upon in devastating detail. Sports columnists for both papers excoriated the university for the coarseness of the drill during which Wheeler expired, for the inadequacy of the medical resources brought to bear on his fatal asthma attack, and for callousness and cynicism in litigation mode. Of course, this coverage didn't change the outcome of a monetary settlement, which a judge imposed on a bereaved mother who'd insisted, to no avail, on her day in court. But it did show, at least, that the news media had a pulse when it came to critical examination of football world and its excesses.

By the time Ted Agu died in 2014, that dynamic no longer obtained. The local daily newspaper, long in decline, was now a virtual zombie institution. Sports sections like those of the *San Francisco Chronicle* still recapped and analyzed the games most of their readers had already watched and read background about online. Sports commentators still provided color and insider insight, and also still heartily weighed in on culture war topics, such as the controversy over the San Francisco 49ers' Colin Kaepernick's protest of going to a knee during the playing of the national anthem, instead of standing respectfully, to protest police violence against Blacks. But tough reporting on college football scandals in all their intricacy was largely out of bounds. Perhaps the reason for this is that the sports department is one of the few vestiges of the classic newspaper format holding much hope for still being a profit center. In the process, local sports franchises, already sacred cows, became almost untouchable.

Against this backdrop, as the University of California carried out its cover-up, the *Chronicle* sprang into action . . . not. No sports columnist there ever commented on the Agu death. (Nor, for that matter, did the newspaper's general editorial page.) What happened, when Cal's multimillion-dollar exposure for a negligent death in football conditioning reached its legal denouement, was that the story got farmed out to the already stretched news department. The mission of the same shrinking staff of reporters there also included taking stock of every question of possible malfeasance or misuse of public funds surrounding the ten-campus UC and its two sister lower tiers of the state's vast higher education system. (They especially liked writing about the bloated size of the administration and their exorbitant salaries.) Therefore — and not without logic — the Agu story was as much or more part of the beat of the *Chronicle*'s higher education reporter as it was that of sportswriters.

With their much more limited knowledge of the story's main players in the football program and the athletic department, the news-side people did what they must have thought was their best to account for the expenditure of $4.75 million in public funds to settle the death of a football player under curious circumstances.

Early in 2016, with a settlement imminent in *Agu v. UC Regents*, the *Chronicle* came in possession of a batch of deposition transcripts. The newspaper's resulting story identified the source of this trove as the Investigative Reporting Program at Cal's Graduate School of Journalism. The director of the program, Lowell Bergman, was the legendary journalist and former *60 Minutes* producer who was portrayed by Al Pacino in *The Insider*, the movie about tobacco industry scandals.[*]

The upshot was a January 29, 2016, article in the *Chronicle* under the headline "UC admits liability in 2014 death of Cal football player." It was the lead story on page 1 on a Saturday, the lowest-circulation day of the week. This would be the one and only item of any depth on the Agu narrative, ever, in this or any other newspaper.

The *Chronicle* headline was mistaken, though only in a trivial, legalistic sense. The university never, technically, "admitted liability" — defendants almost never do in civil settlements, which usually include ritual language

---

[*] Several months later, from a source I won't name, I also acquired a raft of deposition transcripts, some of which I published in their entirety at my website, and all of which were reproduced later in an ebook. My reporting suggests, with near certainty, that this was exactly the same material previously furnished to the *Chronicle*, yet shared with its readers only in a slapdash, cherry-picking manner. Unquestionably, the newspaper published only skewed and incomplete citations to the explosive material therein.

disavowing any such admission. The eventual *Agu v. UC Regents* settlement agreement was careful to include this disclaimer. But it's true that at the time of the article UC was on the verge of forging a significant monetary agreement to end the family's lawsuit; thus, in layperson's shorthand, it was admitting liability.

Nit-picking the headline is the least of the problems with the *Chronicle* coverage. While the story made clear that something awful had happened, and that the degrees of awfulness included aspects of poor handling of Agu's sickle cell trait on that fateful morning on a campus hillside, the article soft-pedaled or altogether ignored the university's urgent and ongoing cover-up methods. At that point the reporters may not have had their hands on many, or any, of the documents later produced in my Public Records Act case. But they still had plenty of damning material, and they left almost all of it on the cutting-room floor. The deposition transcripts, for example, laid out both Batten's obstructive phone call to Beaver and the former's stammering response when he was asked to account for it under oath. In reading the *Chronicle*'s unfocused version of the narrative, as much or more outrage would have been generated by such details as the paucity of grievance counseling resources for Agu's teammates in the following hours and days.

The journalism craft has a saying for what the *San Francisco Chronicle* served up here. It was a clinic in "burying the lead."

When I asked the Cal journalism school's Bergman about this, he offered no real defense. "While we provided certain information and editorial guidance the reporting and editing was done by a Chronicle writer and editor," Bergman emailed me. Bergman's response (before he cut off communication with me) came down to something along the lines of, *We consulted good, but they wrote bad.*

Michael Gray, then the *Chronicle*'s editor for enterprise and investigations, fared no better. "I believe [our story] presented an accurate account of the pertinent events leading up to and following Ted Agu's death," Gray emailed me. ". . . It doesn't appear that you are suggesting there was any error in the Ted Agu story, just that you believe it did not contain certain information you believe might be pertinent."

Yes, that's one way to put it.

The family's wrongful death lawsuit settlement was finalized in April 2016. Ambrose and Emilia Agu, Ted's parents, and one of their lawyers, Steve Yerrid, did an exit interview on ESPN's investigative program, *Outside the Lines*. The Agus wondered how the University of California, to which they'd entrusted their son *in loco parentis*, could have so fumbled his care and well-being. Then, they went away.

In the late spring of 2016, with the family settlement in the books, an uproar ensued when Cal faculty critics of the athletic department exposed the Tanji-Murray "review" of the football strength and conditioning program as a sham. The document was conflicted, cursory, unprofessional — an embarrassment.

Cal chancellor Nicholas Dirks, in the last lap of a four-year tenure strewn with scandals in several areas, not just athletics, responded by announcing that the university would commission a second and better report on football strength and conditioning. The media kerfuffle subsided.

What Dirks wound up actually doing — and not until five months later, in November, when no one any longer was closely watching — proved as effective as it was sneaky. For Review 2.0, Cal tapped Dr. Elizabeth Joy, past president of the American College of Sports Medicine, and Wayne Brazil, a retired Berkeley law professor who was known for a mediation business. But unbeknownst to the public, Dirks had changed the charging instructions. Joy and Brazil were asked to compose a rendering of what would be best practices for a contemporary college football strength and conditioning program. The authors of the report were told to remain resolutely forward-looking and academic in their approach; there was to be no retrospective investigation or evaluation of the events of 2013–14.

Whereas Review 1.0 had been a sloppy, rigged investigation, Review 2.0 was a professional compendium of sound recommendations — but also no investigation at all. Just to make sure any possible remaining sense of accountability would be beaten into submission, the Joy-Brazil report, after passing through multiple hands for tweaks and revisions, would not get finalized and published for another 17 months, in April 2018.

As it happened, during the previous winter's Cal football conditioning there had been a scary echo of the Ted Agu incident. That story starts in October 2017, when an African-American sophomore player was pulled out of practice because he was having trouble breathing. It's possible he was laboring due only to the foul air caused by that season's historically severe California wildfires, but with a sickling death in their immediate recent history, the coaching, training, and medical staffs were disinclined to take any chances. After being sidelined, this student stayed active, doing light workouts on his own, before returning to the full team's winter conditioning on January 16, 2018. He told the staff that his work in the intervening months had been limited by nagging lower back pain.

On January 16, 2018, the newly regathered team did an intense session of circuit weightlifting. The session lasted about 90 minutes, including breaks, with rapid repetitions of bench presses, planks, and squats, and fast transitions between stations. Near the end of this workout, the returning player's lower back pain worsened, with the right side becoming more acute than the left; it was the first time he'd experienced such pain on the right. Team sources said the player wondered at the time whether he might be enduring a sickling episode. (He was a sickle cell trait carrier. It's not known how many identified carriers were on the Cal squad in that year's round of non-mandatory screening.)

Afterward, in the training room, still enduring low-back pain, the player became dizzy and vomited. Though his vital signs were stable and he was alert and talking, the staff called 911. He was hospitalized two nights with what was diagnosed as "non-traumatic rhabdomyolysis." Upon release, the player gradually transitioned back to full team activities and even played in the spring intrasquad game.

Asked about the January 2018 incident when my reporting brought it to light half a year later, the university issued this statement: "We are not able to respond to this request for personal medical information without violating federal laws that protect the privacy and confidentiality of student medical records. The health and safety of our student-athletes is our highest priority, and Cal Athletics and Cal Sports Medicine adhere to best practices on medical matters."

Like the general in that old saying, the University of California, Berkeley, could be proud of having made the necessary adjustments for "fighting the last war."

Thomas R. Beaver, M.D.
Forensic Pathologist
56639 Overseas Highway
Marathon, FL 33050
305-743-9011
916-850-9578

The Honorable Gregory J. Ahern   August 7, 2015
Alameda County Sheriff/Coroner
2901 Peralta Oaks Ct.
2nd Floor
Oakland, CA 94605

Dear Sheriff Ahern:

As you know, I performed the initial autopsy on Ted Agu. Initially, based on the information available to me at that time, I believed the cause of death was best certified as Hypertrophic Cardiomyopathy. However, after I resigned as the Chief Forensic Pathologist for the Alameda County Sheriff's Office, I discovered material and highly significant facts concerning Ted Agu's death that have changed my opinion. Based upon this information, that contradicts the initial information I received indicating this was an immediate and instantaneous death, it is clear to me that Ted Agu died from sickling crisis relating to his sickle cell trait. His death was not instantaneous nor was it related to hypertrophic cardiomyopathy. It is very important (for the family and otherwise) to determine an accurate cause of death. Therefore, I feel obligated to formally request the Coroner's findings regarding Ted Agu's cause of death be amended.

Recently, I gave a deposition in the pending litigation between Ted Agu's family and the University of California Berkeley. I have enclosed a copy of this deposition for your review. My sworn testimony sets forth, in detail, the basis and reasons for my opinion regarding the cause of his premature death.

A brief summary of my testimony might be helpful. When I initially examined Mr. Agu's body, it was pristine. The only thing I noticed was that his heart was mildly enlarged. However, the enlargement was very slight and was close to normal, given that he was a rather large athlete. Even at that time, I felt the condition was not as significant as I would have expected for it to be the cause of this death. Shortly after I examined the body, I received a phone call from Dr. Batten, the team physician for the University of California's football team. Dr. Batten told me that Mr. Agu was "doing fine" during the football conditioning drill and that he suddenly collapsed and died. He further told me that it was his view that Ted Agu's death was a cardiac event.

Only later, when I received and reviewed the microscopic slides, I appreciated a significant amount of sickled red blood cells throughout Mr. Agu's tissues. Certainly, the amount of sickling I observed was enough to cause death. At this point, I had two potential causes of death – hypertrophic cardiomyopathy and sickling crisis. Based on what Dr. Batten told me, as well as the only information I had, was that Ted Agu had died suddenly. The clinical presentation of a death is often extremely important in determining an accurate cause of death. A sudden death with instantaneous collapse is consistent with a cardiac event not sickle cell crisis. At the time of the autopsy report, the only information I had was that the onset of symptoms was sudden and instantaneous. This led to my initial conclusion. However, I remained concerned by the amount of sickling I saw in this young man's tissues, and the autopsy report specifically references this point. In the report, I clearly state that my initial opinion was "based upon information available to me at the time (emphasis added)." My intent was to leave room for a new cause of death if additional facts were discovered.

I have now reviewed numerous sworn depositions given by University of California football players who were present at the workout the morning Mr. Agu died and who actually witnessed the extent of his struggles prior to his final collapse. These players' sworn testimony makes one critical fact very clear – Ted Agu did not die suddenly. Instead, he had significant difficulty during the conditioning drill for many minutes before he collapsed. Contrary to the initial information I was given, Mr. Agu's condition gradually got worse over a number of minutes as the drill progressed. The drill required the players to run ten times up and down a steep hill. The testimony reflects that the decedent started having difficulty around the 5th or 6th lap, and his condition got worse as each lap progressed, until he finally collapsed on the 10th and final lap.

The overwhelming and convincing information I now have indicates that Ted Agu's death was neither sudden nor immediate. On the contrary, the events of that day are inconsistent with a cardiac death and instead, reflect a sickling death. As noted above, Mr. Agu's heart was at best, mildly "enlarged" for an athlete his size. However, the extent of the sickling in his body was quite significant.

Based upon the events that occurred prior to his death and as the forensic pathologist who personally performed the autopsy on Mr. Agu, I respectfully submit that the death certificate should be amended to state the cause of death as: Acute Sickle Cell Crisis. The manner of death remains natural. If needed, I welcome the opportunity to take any further steps necessary to ensure that the accurate cause of death be reflected in an amended Coroner's Report and an amended Death Certificate. In view of the family's loss, this valid and accurate cause of death needs to be incorporated into the official public records as soon as possible.

Please feel free to contact me if I may be of any assistance in this matter.

Respectfully submitted,

Thomas R. Beaver, M.D.

CHAPTER 4

Litigating the University of California's Ted Agu Death Cover-Up

The federal Freedom of Information Act (FOIA) and its state counterparts — in California it's called the California Public Records Act (CPRA or "see-prah") — are imperfect vehicles for fulfilling the goals of government and public agency openness in a democratic society. Of all the practical obstacles to the ideals of public information law through CPRA, the main one is the simple truth that knowledge is power. In these fights, public agencies always hold all the cards: they know what they have and what they don't. Citizens and journalists seeking CPRA compliance are flying blind. To a large extent and almost by definition, public records requesters can be accused of being on fishing expeditions when they seek specific information supporting investigations of possible official malfeasance.

Throughout 2016, while investigating the stories of the Ted Agu death and the Ted Agu death cover-up, I made a series of requests under CPRA to the University of California, Berkeley, the University of California, Davis, and the overall University of California system's central Office of the President. What I got in return was a mix of fragments of document releases complying with my requests and, most revealingly, clever delays and stonewalling.

Some of the material eventually produced was substantial, on point, and eye-opening. Per that Mark Twain adage about how the truth is slow to get dressed for battle against already baked-in lies, the new information was also conveniently late.

My reporting strongly suggested these productions were incomplete. In certain instances, reporting not only suggested incompleteness but established it. An example was my independent acquisition of Damon Harrington's "Winter Workout Contract," with its outline of the "Grave Digger" and other punishment drills. The university claimed to have no record of such a document.

By the time my pas de deux with UC through the California judicial system ended years later, there were more than 100 pages of other documents leaked to me by campus sources, yet officially denied by the university as having existed at all; or, if their existence was grudgingly acknowledged, claimed to being not subject to public records release because of one legal exemption or another. And there were still other documents blocked from official and full disclosure by baroque arguments enabled by a judge who also happened to be both a UC Berkeley college and law school alumnus. The collective internal resources and judicial bias brought to bear on covering up the circumstances and management of a football death took on the state equivalent of national security secrets, and had similar overtones of the games people play to protect them.

My CPRA case largely turned on a failure to enforce one of the core requirements of the statute. This law's plain language contains at least a token mindfulness of the problem that only the public agency knows what it has, and that the expectations of and burdens on the parties must be apportioned accordingly. Specifically, CPRA builds into its practical operation a provision that the public agency must work with the public records requester to make requests "focused and effective."

This rule proves to be as unenforced as it's nice. In my own scenario, whenever there was a question or problem, Cal and its sister entities simply decreed that they'd fully supplied all relevant documents (or claimed that the sum of such documents was zero). They could get away with this conduct because judicial oversight of the "focused and effective" requirement is toothless to the point of meaninglessness. Under our legal system, the rest proceeds to get whittled to a toothpick by the experienced and well-rehearsed maneuverings of the University of California's large staff of defense lawyers. At no point and at no level did the state courts show any spine when it came to holding the public agency's recalcitrance against it.

At the University of California Office of the President, at least 70 full-time attorneys hold forth, almost all with six-figure salaries. (This doesn't include the outside law firms brought in to co-counsel on big-ticket matters like the Agu wrongful death lawsuit.) These worthies are supported by dozens more clerks and secretaries. Of course, a large, complex entity needs a competent legal department, and in many situations it needs vigorous advocacy. Unfortunately, in the CPRA environment, legalistic defense can be offensive to the public interest. At key moments, the university's tactics are sharp, at odds with the educational mission, and even actionably unethical.

One senior counsel, Michael R. Goldstein, did more than just orchestrate delays and evasions in my quest for revealing documents; in sworn declarations to the court, he also committed serial, unambiguous, and effective unindicted perjury. The courts never laid a glove on the university for its bad faith and blatant lies. As this book was headed for publication, I submitted to the state bar association an exhaustive complaint of attorney misconduct against Goldstein, for violations of the code of conduct in the areas of "dishonesty, fraud, deceit, or reckless or intentional misrepresentation" and "conduct that is prejudicial to the administration of justice" (respectively, Rules 8.4(c) and (d)).

After Ted Agu died, Dr. Casey Batten obstructed justice and manipulated the coroner into a false finding that the cause was heart disease. And Batten's punishment was a successful move up to the Los Angeles Rams. After Michael Goldstein was finished defending litigation aimed at finding out more about the cover-up actions of Batten and others, Goldstein similarly went on to his next case and his next paycheck, courtesy of California taxpayers and UC tuition-payers.

The stage was set for slugging things out in court after December 15, 2016, when Cal's public records coordinator, Liane Ko, emailed me 46 pages of partially redacted reproductions of emails among various officials. Ko's cover message wrapped things up: "The release of these documents completes this records request, and we now consider this request closed."

Now nearly a year into a CPRA request process I knew to be incomplete, and with no effort by the university on the "focused and effective" front, the only relief would come from a petition in state court to compel full compliance. Toward that end, I retained San Francisco attorney and old friend Roy S. Gordet, whose main practice area was intellectual property but who'd done a quick study of public information litigation while representing me, successfully, in a FOIA against the Department of Homeland Security.*

On March 24, 2017, Gordet sent on my behalf a letter to the campus PRA office reiterating my outstanding concerns. In legal terms, this letter put the university on "constructive notice."

On April 18, we filed *Muchnick v. UC Regents* at the Superior Court in Alameda County. Litigation would drag on through 2022. At Superior Court, I lost almost every motion, in several instances under circumstances I found exceedingly shady. Yet in the end the court *did* rule that the release of hundreds of pages of resulting new documents had to be credited, under CPRA, to my action in suing and to Gordet's painstaking and years-long advocacy. Governing this decision was a doctrine of case law called "catalyst theory." Hanging in for years of David-v.-Goliath legal battles triggered court orders pegged to various negotiated categories and structures of production, making me "the prevailing party." Even Judge Jeffrey S. Brand, who'd ruled so frustratingly against us in numerous other motions, agreed.

Brand's decision didn't hold up. On order of the court, the two sides negotiated the payment of the prevailing party's legal fees, and agreed on Gordet's discounted figure of $125,000. Before the final court judgment could be entered, though, the university appealed to the First District Court

---

* That case, for immigration records of serial sex criminal George Gibney, a former Irish Olympic swim coach, settled at the Ninth Circuit Court of Appeals.

of Appeal. There, in an extraordinary twist, a three-judge panel reversed the discretionary finding of the lower court judge and concluded that I was the losing, not winning, party. From Gordet's standpoint, this reversal had material consequences, as it meant he wouldn't get compensated for the risks he'd taken in logging hundreds of hours of work.

For me, the Court of Appeal outcome was inconsequential; I'd gotten my hands on the documents I'd gotten, and not gotten those I hadn't. The designation of prevailing party was more about bragging rights than anything substantive.

The hardball UC played in order to so "win" was as revealing as the root Agu death cover-up itself. As far as I was concerned, in withholding for years what should have been immediately produced public information, the university already had succeeded in its aims, as a practical matter. That is, it had obscured and diluted widespread understanding of what had taken place at Berkeley in connection with the Agu death. That event was now remote disputed history, not widely received and consensually accepted news. Ted *who*?

But UC's legal eagles weren't content to stop there. In proceeding to pound home pernicious CPRA practices and bad legal precedents, they sent the additional message to anyone out there that this institution would stop at little to dodge accountability for its fealty to football world, and would go so far as to seek to cripple and intimidate critics positioned to expose associated wrongdoing.

Welcome to the sausage factory of the California Public Records Act. Along with the intermittent happy ending, this cottage industry also produces vats of truth-dodging legal pork, plus mountains of rainforest-denuding paper.

On June 5, 2017, Roy Gordet and I had our first "meet and confer" with the UC legal team since the filing of the CPRA lawsuit. The meeting was at Office of the President headquarters in Oakland. In attendance were Michael Goldstein, the senior counsel, and Liane Ko, the Berkeley campus CPRA compliance coordinator.

One of the first things I said to Goldstein at this meeting was, "If you had an issue with or questions about my requests, didn't the law require you to work with the requester to make his efforts 'focused and effective,' before we had to sue?"

Goldstein's reply was glib: "Well, isn't that exactly what we're doing here?"

Of course, "here" was after I'd already hired a lawyer and gone to the trouble and expense of filing a lawsuit. Goldstein's edgy answer was consistent with an ongoing strategy whereby UC leveraged its asymmetrical resources and legal firepower for the purpose of wearing down a nosy journalist.

What emerged from the meeting was an agreement that our side would submit a list of search terms — "Agu death" and so forth — which would be cross-referenced with the email and other document archives matching the names of key administrators. This "algorithm search," as Goldstein called it, would be used to re-check whether there were any other documents eligible for CPRA release that had previously slipped through the cracks.

This process wound up taking months, involving what Goldstein would call "Phase 1," "Phase 2," and "follow-up." On October 17, 2017, Goldstein let us know the outcome of the vaunted algorithm search: "We have identified no responsive non-exempt records other than those we have already released."

This stalemate took us into the area of public information law called the "Vaughn Index." This term was rooted in a federal FOIA case involving a party named Vaughn, and the law has become the gold standard in both federal and state public records cases. In a Vaughn Index, the public agency withholding documents on claims of various exemptions (for example, the need not to compromise a still-pending criminal investigation) must file with the court a complete listing with descriptions of the individual documents and their corresponding exemption claims. Other types of cases propound what are called privilege logs to list documents protected by attorney-client privilege and other forms of confidentiality. Essentially, a Vaughn Index is a special kind of privilege log. It forces the withholding party to do more than just make a blanket claim that what it has produced to date was the complete and proper response. A Vaughn meant UC would have to put up more about what it had shut up.

The university resisted doing a Vaughn Index. Its rationale utterly mystified one judge, yet would be blessed by a second one.

In digging in its heels, UC relied on a 1974 federal law, the Family Educational Rights and Privacy Act. Also sometimes referred to as the Buckley Amendment (after its author, Senator James Buckley of New York), FERPA restricts the ability of educational institutions to release information about students.

FERPA is actually a narrow statute that was designed for policies or practices in securing particular centrally maintained educational records. More than 20 years ago, the U.S. Supreme Court rejected an expansive definition of "educational records" and said that for FERPA purposes, the term applied only to those held in a central repository. For reference to the potential disclosure of sensitive or protected documents concerning individual students, the FERPA argument had minimum plausibility in *Muchnick v. UC Regents*. And even that angle was rendered moot with respect to Ted Agu, who was dead and, under law clarified by a letter released by the U.S. Department of Education, no longer could claim privacy rights. In reference to the task of assembling a mere *index* to show what the university had in its possession but would not agree to produce in our CPRA lawsuit, for whatever reason, the FERPA defense was less than implausible; it made no sense at all.

It's easy to do a thought experiment showing how, in the universe of intercollegiate sports, holding up FERPA as some sort of all-encompassing privacy mandate is a *reductio ad absurdum*. NCAA FERPing could lead to such outcomes as not facilitating media coverage of football games — after all, the public has no "right" to intrude into knowledge of the names, ages, heights, weights, high school backgrounds, and statistics of the players. We can presume the schools profiting from football world, for which publicity drives massive revenues, would never go for *that*.

During the COVID-19 pandemic, the University of Alabama cited FERPA to refuse to disclose to the public the number of infections at the school from the virus, and even banned faculty from speaking about the subject on campus. UC's gambit in the Agu death was in line with new legal efforts by universities across the country to abuse FERPA as a wide-ranging fig leaf for hiding credible allegations of malfeasance.

By now, we were up to fall 2017, thanks to UC's delays and court extensions for filing its basic answer to our complaint. At a hearing, our judge, Kimberly E. Colwell, expressed extreme skepticism of the position that a Vaughn Index could be suppressed merely because of the university's assertion that my records requests had triggered FERPA by name-checking specific student-athletes (Fabiano Hale, J.D. Hinnant, and Joey Mahalic, as well as Agu).

Judge Colwell's skepticism only hardened when she quizzed Goldstein at the hearing. She asked him to offer at least a ballpark idea of how much overall material we were talking about here. Three pages' worth of documents? Three thousand? Goldstein said he was barred from answering even that question — because of FERPA.

The judge replied that she did not see it that way and had never heard of such a legal doctrine, and was poised to order a Vaughn Index. She added, however, that she preferred not to make snap rulings from the bench on important issues. "I'll order briefing," Colwell said.

The university filed a "motion to protect" and we responded. We were feeling pretty good about the direction of the case. That's when the judicial system served up its first major curveball. One day we looked up to find that the Superior Court had reassigned the case away from Judge Colwell. We were never told why.

Now, I hasten to add that I have no evidence that the sidelining of Kimberly Colwell was anything other than a routine caseload management move by the presiding judge (Alameda County has more than 60 judges). By the same token, I can't say with any confidence that Colwell's disappearance wasn't other than routine — even highly irregular or corrupt. All I know for sure is that when UC's kooky motion to get out of doing a Vaughn Index landed, the decider was no longer Colwell. Instead, it was Judge Brand, retired dean of the law school at the University of San Francisco, and a graduate of both Cal's College of Letters & Science and the Boalt School of Law (now Berkeley Law).

Brand proceeded to swallow his alma mater's global interpretation of FERPA as a bar to the standard public information law protocol of a Vaughn Index. In its place, the new judge did order a custom-made alternative. He called this a "framework" of "categories" of withheld documents. Later, this would prove important, when the Court of Appeal, out of nowhere, would reverse Brand's finding that his precious "categories" fell under the commonly held theory that my lawsuit had catalyzed the release of new public records. The appellate justices would have had a much harder time pulling off their stunt in the face of a classic Vaughn Index, rather than a flimsily defined "framework."

At the same time he found in UC's favor in the motion to protect from doing an honest-to-goodness Vaughn Index, Brand sent the parties back to meet and confer on the construction of appropriate categories that the court felt would tiptoe around UC's relief.

While this ruling was intellectually silly, the upshot of an alternative "categories" structure — which I came to regard as something of a Rube Goldberg device — did, at least, add up to qualified good news for fans of transparency. And beginning nearly a year later, in September 2018, UC did indeed spin out a series of new document productions. The first release, 194 pages in all, contained 48 pages of internal emails on such important topics as the sports information office's prepping of Dr. Batten and others on what to say at the media briefing held hours after Agu died. It was now provable, for example, that Batten had been scripted to say: "Our hearts are heavy. . . . What I can say at this time is . . . " — and then to lay down a false narrative of when Agu was stricken, and in response to the most obvious questions, to assert that privacy concerns precluded confirming that he had a pre-existing medical condition. (And all this, remember, while the doctor behind the scenes was *concealing* Agu's sickle cell trait from county medical examiner Beaver, and steering him toward a finding of heart disease.)

As also was developed in the previous chapter, this email cache exposed the obsessive monitoring by athletic department executives of online discussion board mentions of sickle cell trait. Accompanying the monitoring was an organized effort to tamp down any such references.

A second batch of UC records production from the Judge Brand–ordered Vaughn Index–substitute "framework," later in September 2018, totaled nearly 400 pages. These consisted of heavily redacted emails between and among Cal officials. Almost nothing there was unmasked except for the names of senders and recipients, the subject lines, and the names of attachment files. Even so, these documents contributed substantially to the narratives of the anticipation of the coroner's findings and of communications laying the groundwork for approval of the Agu family's $4.75 million lawsuit settlement. (The emails showed that approval of the settlement by the board of regents was orchestrated for an "interim" meeting between regularly calendared meetings — perhaps for the purpose of keeping the event out of public view. That is what often happens in the resolution of the university's major pieces of litigation.)

We weren't done. A new battle involved my effort to uncover campus police records in the Agu death. As noted earlier, the existence of 141 pages of police reports emerged from the family lawsuit, where discovery and deposition testimony also revealed that a super-majority of those pages weren't forwarded to the Alameda County sheriff. Yet in response in my CPRA case, Cal produced none of them. In its "framework" productions, there wasn't a word about police reports. We kept asking about them and we kept getting variations on the answer, "What police reports? What are you talking about?"*

At a hearing before Judge Brand, Goldstein finally conceded that what we seemed to be referring to was what he called a particular "binder" of

---

* Earlier, the Berkeley CPRA compliance office had sent me the police report on J.D. Hinnant's attack on Fabiano Hale, three months before the Agu death — but, curiously, only after the report had already been requested by and released to the campus newspaper, the *Daily Cal*, which proceeded to do nothing with the information. (Across time, the *Daily Cal* would publish two op-ed page essays by me summarizing my own ongoing reporting and analysis. A third opinion article got accepted by the editors, then censored from publication at the last minute on the grounds that they feared a lawsuit by the university if they so much as published my opinion that the football program's commercial considerations often trumped doing the right thing. Readers can view the censored article at my website, https://concussioninc.net/?p=13789.)

police reports. UC claimed that the binder contents were exempt from disclosure. This couldn't be because of FERPA — that federal statute specifically excluded police records from privacy protection. California's CPRA, however, did exempt certain types of investigatory records. Bottom line, we'd have to plead another court motion in order to figure out what was what.

The Berkeley campus police department came to this issue with considerable credibility problems. There was Lieutenant DeCoulode's PR blocking in front of Sonny Dykes in the early days after the Hinnant criminal assault of Hale, when the local media were still somewhat focused on nefariousness in Cal football and the cop was asserting to them that the altercation had nothing to do with the head coach. There was Detective Bennigson's softball interrogation of conditioning coach Harrington — followed by the do-over interview, with blatant prompting and rehearsal of answers seemingly designed to put the sickle cell trait issue to bed, for which DeCoulode joined Bennigson and directed him. And thanks to the two earlier email document productions in the CPRA litigation, there was the profile of the campus police chief, Margo Bennett, who could be accused of having put less emphasis on public safety than she did on the PR agendas of her bosses.

In the previous chapter, Bennett in March 2014 was seen emailing vice chancellor John Wilton with a warning not to share with others a batch of documents she'd given him the day before. Bennett explained to Wilton that "the case" was "not available for a PRA request and I'd like to keep it that way." (*What* case?)

On April 21, 2014, in an email discussion of the Agu cause of death, Wilton wrote to Bennett: "I wonder if we should bring Dan M into the picture?" Dan M was Dan Mogulof, assistant vice chancellor for executive communications — the chief of media relations. To be very clear, the "From" line of the email read: "John Wilton." The "To" line read: "Margo BENNETT; Ann JEFFREY."

When we pointed all this out to the court, Bennett countered with a sworn statement breaking new ludicrous ground. "Mr. Muchnick is in error," the chief declared, when "he implies that Mr. Wilton's question was directed to me." Of course, my declaration had "implied" nothing; it had stated, flatly and accurately, that the email was sent from Wilton to Bennett, and I reproduced it. "I was updating him as part of my responsibilities as his direct report. His email concerning Mr. Mogulof was directed to his Chief of Staff [Ann Jeffrey], not to me." Typically for the hearsay that Goldstein and his boss, UC general counsel and vice president for legal affairs Charles F. Robinson, lobbed up throughout the case, Bennett didn't explain why she, the recipient, rather than Wilton, the sender, was the one testifying as to what Wilton intended by sending the email to Margo Bennett, first, and Ann Jeffrey, second.

When it came time to decide whether the 141 pages of the police binder would be daylighted, Brand reprised his deference to the university, with little regard for the rigor of the arguments on both sides. On November 18, 2018, he issued a "tentative decision" taking tentativeness to new levels. "The motion of petitioner Muchnick to require the Regents to disclose a 141 page police report relating to the death of Ted Agu is UNDECIDED," Brand thundered.

In the supporting commentary as to why he'd be further agonizing over a final decision, the judge signaled just where he believed UC had fallen short. Dutifully, the university had already supplied a declaration by Chief Bennett asserting that it was Berkeley campus policy "that when a police officer responds to an incident, then it becomes a police matter," in Brand's paraphrase. (So, when a football player collapses dead in a conditioning drill, it's a police matter, by "policy." Likewise, when an 80-year-old emeritus professor collapses dead in his office, it's a police matter, by "policy.")

Additionally, Detective Bennigson swore that the campus police performed due diligence for every campus-located fatality. The cops investigate "all deaths, whether by natural cause, suicide, homicide, or otherwise," Brand observed, and with a detective correspondingly assigned.

The problem with this position, the judge pointed out, was that the court didn't just need affirmation that deaths were in the jurisdiction and job description of the campus police. In order to qualify for one of the CPRA exemptions from public release, a public agency must bring to the table more than "bare assertion that it relates to investigation"; more than "solely by presenting evidence that the police collected the information and/or conducted the investigation." CPRA case law established that there must be a further showing of an investigation *with the purpose of determining whether a violation of law may occur or has occurred*. Again, not just an investigation conducted in whole or in part by police officers, but a *particular type of investigation* — one of criminal activity.

Plainly, the university had failed to justify keeping the police binder under wraps: Brand wrote he was "not persuaded" by an "implicit argument that the investigation was a law enforcement investigation because any death raises a reasonable suspicion of criminal activity."

Still, Brand went on to muse, there were "plausible" rationales for secrecy that so far remained unarticulated by UC. One might be "reasonable suspicion of criminal activity," such as that used by a police officer to detain a person. Another might be "probable cause," such as that used to back up an application for a search warrant. A third might be a particular investigation's "dominant purpose."

Apparently determined to remain "undecided" until such time as he had enough ammunition to decide against me, the judge now ordered "supplemental" briefing to clarify the issue that was bothering him.

Brand's tentative decision to nowhere was nothing less than a road map to exactly what UC needed to do in supplemental briefing in order to cure, for the judge's purposes, its flawed contention that the law supported keeping the disputed 141-page police binder out of my hands. The UC general counsel's office didn't miss the cue; it proceeded, note by note, to do just that.

The court issued its final ruling in early 2019: the university "has demonstrated that the Department's investigation of the death of Ted Agu was a law enforcement investigation for purposes of the Govt Code 6254(f) exemption for 'investigations conducted by . . . any state or local police agency.'" Our motion to compel release of the 141-page campus police binder was denied.

This loss on the court motion became somewhat moot when I proceeded to acquire the full contents of the police binder, anyway, via a campus source, and was able to report further on the evidence there of

Chief Bennett's and her department's collusion with the Berkeley administration in tamping down knowledge that Agu died from an exertional
attack associated with sickle cell trait.

On March 29, 2019 — now nearly two years in — UC senior counsel
Goldstein emailed my attorney, Gordet, to pass along two afterthought
documents. The university had "inadvertently" failed to include them in
previous productions, Goldstein explained.

These were an email exchange between Dr. Casey Batten, the Cal
football team physician, and Christopher Patti, the chief campus counsel.
The bodies of the emails were entirely redacted on a claim of attorney-
client privilege. The one from Patti to Batten was dated December 4,
2015, with the subject line "Agu Case." The one from Batten to Patti was
dated December 15, 2015, with the subject line "ATTORNEY CLIENT
PRIVILEGED COMMUNICATION," and with an attachment file whose
name was redacted.

December 2015 was the period after the deposition testimony of the
coroner office's Beaver in the Agu family lawsuit exposed Batten's inap-
propriate call to him and the inaccurate initial finding that Agu had died of
hypertrophic cardiomyopathy, rather than exertional sickling.

Judge Jeffrey S. Brand saved his best and most linguistically tortured gift to
his alma mater for last. This was a ruling that a lengthy thread of emails
among Cal administrators discussing the Ted Agu death didn't have to be
released, despite the record showing that a deputy athletic director had
already forwarded the entire thread to his father, an outsider.

The deputy AD was one Solly Fulp, part of the chain of Cal authorities
whom backup quarterback Joey Mahalic, a whistleblower of Damon
Harrington's toxic strength and conditioning regime, had consulted before
talking to the campus police.

Fulp's email faux pas showed that, like many of us from time to time,
he was an imperfect keeper of secrets. Fulp was and is, additionally, a

skillful maintainer of his status as a mover and shaker in the college sports-industrial complex.

In June 2014, four months after the Agu death, Chancellor Dirks announced that athletic director Sandy Barbour was leaving her position "to accept a new role on campus." Thus began jockeying among the deputies to be chosen as her successor. Dirks named one of them, Mike Williams, the interim AD. In the fall, a search committee was formed for the hire of the permanent replacement. Fulp was one of the six leading candidates, too, but Williams won out. (By then, Barbour had skipped to the AD post at Penn State.)

Fulp landed himself a nice consolation prize. Wilton, the vice chancellor for finance, was creating a new central administration position to oversee what was being called the University Partnership Program. The website for the program explained that the UPP was a platform for "meaningful, campuswide relationships with partners by collaborating across units to create partnership opportunities that align with Berkeley's values and mission of teaching, research and public service." What this gobbledygook added up to was that Cal henceforth would have a highly paid administrator solely dedicated to the recruitment and servicing of corporate sponsors. (At the time of this book's publication, UPP partners included Bank of the West, Peet's Coffee, PepsiCo, and Farmers Insurance.)

To save money, the university didn't hire an outside firm to conduct a search for the new boss of UPP. And to save time, the opening for "Executive Director of University Business Partnerships and Services" was listed only for the minimum two weeks required by federal law. At the end of this clearly rigged process, Solly Fulp landed his new post at Cal carrying an annual salary of $230,000. Even though it was just a one-year contract, the university threw in a $50,000 "signing bonus."

One possible explanation for the bonus, bringing the package up to $280,000, was that it was a contrivance to keep Solly Fulp and his family living in the manner to which they'd become accustomed. At the athletic department in 2014, Fulp enjoyed a salary and benefits package potentially totaling $345,178. Included was a $20,000 performance bonus if the Golden Bears football team got invited to a major bowl game (they didn't). Also a

$10,000 bonus if they went to a non-major bowl (nope). Plus a $20,000 tip "for results relative to goal in the new business development area" (maybe!). In addition, the family Fulp were perked membership in Renaissance ClubSport, a high-end fitness facility.

For sums like this, you could procure a lot of Bunsen burners for the chemistry labs.

From his new perch, Fulp worked Berkeley corporate sponsors for two years. He left in 2017 to become senior vice president, then executive vice president, of Learfield, a college sports marketing company. Fulp had worked previously at Learfield, from 2008 to 2011, before joining the Cal athletic department. A revolving door is never the kind that hits you in the butt on the way out.

In our CPRA case, Fulp became a person of interest for attorney Gordet and me because of a newly disclosed batch of emails of Berkeley athletic department and central administration executives and officials. UC had produced these as part of Judge Brand's Rube Goldberg–esque "framework." The contents of the emails were all but completely redacted with a claim of attorney-client privilege. (One or more lawyers were in the "To," "From," or "cc" line in all these messages, justifying the blanket privilege claim.)

One email was not like the others. It was dated April 23, 2014, and it appeared to be a forward of the entire discussion thread. The sender was Solly Fulp. The recipient was "Dad" — most likely Fulp's father, as rendered by a computer email program's autocomplete from the sender's contact list.

We figured out that Solly Fulp's father was named Ian Fulp, and he was a municipal parks and recreation director living in Alaska. "See below," Solly wrote to Dad — followed by the pages-long blacked-out thread.

Why Fulp the younger was sharing confidential and sensitive university communications with Fulp père was unknown. One hypothesis was that Solly might have been idly sharing his work that day, or perhaps the two just had an ongoing and freewheeling dialogue, on email and in real life, regarding Cal Athletics behind the scenes. Regardless, this indiscretion, on its face, torpedoed any claim that the email wasn't a public record. There's a principle in public information law that disclosure to one opens the door to disclosure to all.

We subpoenaed and deposed Solly Fulp. In 2022, Donald Trump took the Fifth Amendment more than 400 times at a deposition by the New York State attorney general. During the House of Representatives January 6 Committee investigation, many Trump aides and associates invoked faulty memories in declining to answer important questions. Fulp's deposition in our case was at a court reporter's office in San Francisco. In the course of one hour, Fulp answered "I cannot recall" and its variations 119 times, by my manual count.

Among the things Solly Fulp couldn't recall were (a) sending the 2014 email; (b) why he sent it; and (c) whether he'd ever had any conversations about Agu with any of the other university officials on the email chain. Oh, and also whether he'd had any conversations about Agu with Ian Fulp (whom Solly did acknowledge to be the "Dad" recipient of the message in question).

Again, we thought we were on rock-solid ground in moving to Judge Brand to unredact the Fulp-to-Dad email on the basis of its already existing disclosure to a member of the public with no professional connection to the University of California. The email, we argued, clearly failed the test for attorney-client privilege.

In rejoinder, the UC general counsel's office threw up their usual little of this and little of that.

And as always, Judge Jeffrey S. Brand had the last word. "The court finds," he wrote in his decision, "that Fulp forwarded the email to his father intending it to be a confidential intra-family communication in the manner of 'Dad, this why I've been so busy at work [sic].'" In so doing, Fulp was not "acting within the scope of his or her membership, agency, office, or employment." He was acting "in his personal capacity and was not acting on behalf of the Regents. . . . There is no indication that Fulp's email to 'dad' was related to his employment."

The motion therefore was "DENIED because the Regents has demonstrated that the Fulp email contained attorney-client information and petitioner has not demonstrated that Fulp was acting within the scope of his membership, agency, office, or employment when he disclosed the email to his father."

Notwithstanding a case history suggesting Judge Brand bled the Cal colors of blue and gold through his august black robe, even he, in the end, couldn't bring himself to declare UC the prevailing party. After all, hundreds of pages of previously withheld documents had been released. Nine out of ten people in a bar, sober or otherwise, would conclude that my lawsuit had caused their release.

But UC lawyer Goldstein had more cards to play. Never averse to leaving behind a polemical overreach, he and his team weren't content with defending against a holding that I was the prevailing party. The university entered a "cross-motion" arguing that my case was "clearly frivolous," entitling *UC* to the recovery of its legal fees and costs from *me*. There's not a single precedent for such a holding in a published CPRA case.

"Where's the frivolity," Gordet asked the court, in our search for deeper answers in the Agu death and for years of going toe to toe with the university over the technicalities? Were the families of dead young athletes across the country slapping their thighs over an investigation of how some of these deaths got covered up?

It was in his motions against our fees, and in favor of his client's counter-fees, that Goldstein brought his full "A" game of arrogance. The arrogance was marinated in blatant prevarication. Throughout the case, Goldstein had written in case management statements and briefs — as well as in a personal declaration sworn on penalty of perjury — alternately that the Regents had first proposed trying to get a privacy waiver from the Agu family, and that I had.

That there was a privacy waiver overture to the Agus and which side had first suggested it were facts, in the first place, utterly irrelevant to the fees issue. The mendacity in Goldstein's exploitation of both sides of this question, Gordet told the court, was "mystifying."

The record toted up four times where Goldstein claimed the waiver was petitioner's idea — and five times where he insisted it was respondent's idea. In the brief dated September 10, 2020, Goldstein outdid himself. One section was captioned "The Agu Family Waiver Was Petitioner's Idea . . ." and there were five assertions of such. But Goldstein also wrote, within the very same document, "Petitioner never followed up on *the Regents' suggestion about obtaining waivers*" (italics added)!

Silent on our pointer to multiple bald-faced lies, and blandly negative on the university's quest for punitive fees against me, Brand at least did agree with Gordet's contention that we were the prevailing party. This was the one and only motion the judge decided our way in years of legal jousting. The judge ordered the parties to negotiate Gordet's fees.

Before the general counsel had to bother requisitioning the UC bursar to cut a check, Goldstein was running to the Court of Appeal. As a general rule, appellate courts show great deference to the lower court; they usually choose not to get involved unless there's reason to believe the trial judge below might have abused his discretion.

Not so here. Our case landed at division 5 of the First District. There, the three-justice panel — chief justice Teri L. Jackson, Mark B. Simons, and Rebecca A. Wiseman — did the university's bidding. They decided that Brand, who'd presided over every detail of the case, got it wrong. Even though hundreds of new pages of documents were produced, they came from the "framework" of "categories" concocted after the judge rejected the standard vehicle of a Vaughn Index. Therefore, not a single new piece of significant information, the appellate panel ruled, could be attributed to the language of my original request for documents "dealing with" investigations of the Agu death. Justice Simons, the author of the opinion — and a former adjunct professor at UC's Hastings College of Law in San Francisco — tied himself into verbal knots in maintaining that his completely fact-based rebuke of Brand amounted to a different "legal standard."

Carrying the torch for Gordet and me at the Court of Appeal was John Derrick, who is recognized as one of the state's top appellate specialists. At the oral argument, Derrick tried to point out that there were clearly elements of the document productions falling within even an ungenerous interpretation of my original records request. One example was police chief Bennett's admonition to Vice Chancellor Wilton not to share with others the batch of documents she'd given him, because "the case" was "not open to a PRA request and I'd like to keep it that way." Another example was all the work product of the sports information office coaching everyone on how to dodge questions about Agu's sickle cell trait.

The justices were having none of it. They didn't even bother to ask Goldstein to rebut Derrick as they gaveled down *Muchnick v. UC Regents*. They refused Derrick's request at least to order a specific lower court review of the case's document productions in relation to the language of the original requests. The public agency "prevailed." The journalist "lost."

Left to history is answering the question of whether the California courts' embarrassing dysfunction, and their disfigurement of the state Public Records Act, make for any way to run a candy store — much less an institution of higher learning.

On November 14, 2022 — while in the middle of a futile ultimate petition to the California Supreme Court to intervene — I submitted to the state bar association my attorney misconduct complaint against Goldstein. I'd resolved to take this step two years earlier, before I knew how the underlying case would turn out. Goldstein's lies were blatant, and so was the damage that lying of this nature does to the putative mission of the state public information regime. What I wanted, simply and above all, was a clear addition to the record. As this book was being published, the bar association had assigned an investigator and begun a process anticipated to take several months.

I wrote: "While defending against my CPRA Petition, Michael Goldstein lied to a California court — non-trivially, proactively, repeatedly. In order to establish as much it is not necessary to hear disputed facts. This is because Mr. Goldstein, with bewildering audacity, himself opportunistically and cyclically asserted, under oath, direct contradictions of the same fact. . . . What is before you is not 'his word against mine'; it is 'his word against his word.'"

The CPRA statute, I concluded, cannot function as intended when petitioners seeking relief in the courts are met "with blatant bad faith and willful falsehood."

I might have added that our finest public universities have no chance of achieving their mission of the search for knowledge and truth when they find themselves in bed with football world.

CHAPTER 5

The
Toughness
Games

L ike all sports in their contemporary incarnations, elite football increas-
ingly relies on science, metrics, and an ultra-professionalized class of
coaches poised to interpret them. Statistical and video study combines with
hyper-modern nutrition, training, and focused skills work (along with, arguably in certain cases, the odd borderline performance-enhancing drug). For
spectators, the new fine-tuned athlete produces plays that routinely drop
the jaw, inspire the awe. At times, appreciation of these isolated displays of
individual athletic brilliance can seem to overshadow the point of the game
itself: how compelling are the pace and flow of the action, which team is
winning and by how much.

Some of the great plays are the types of events that used to be seen a
couple of times a year or even a generation. To the lay football fan's eyes,
displays of great athleticism are most evident in those who handle or catch
the ball on every play. The most discerning observers also can tease out
more, such as the nuances of hand-fighting and leverage, exhibiting more
than brute strength, in the trenches of the interior lines.

Any critic of football who won't concede that the sport has artistry as well as brutality leaves himself open to being held as both not credible and hopelessly ideological. Football is popular for many reasons, and some are good ones. The sport does entertain and it's not devoid of redeeming social value. But do the tradeoffs make sense for universal participation? No.

In history, even the grandest and most popular spectacles run their course or get supplanted. The nation, after all, was once galvanized by heavyweight championship boxing matches. Over the years, passels of dilettantes have celebrated the violence of these bouts as grisly literature, and their mode of combat as the "Sweet Science." The question isn't whether football lacks an equivalent riveting and primal beauty. The question is how long it will take before football gets boxinged into somewhat saner proportion. High schools no longer have boxing teams. They've never had cigarette smoking teams.

Part of football's devolution will be tracked in how preparation for it changes across time. Boxing practice gave us punching bags and shadow movement drills to supplement actual sparring. The hardware of football's contribution to sports civilization included blocking sleds and tackling dummies to supplement scrimmage practice. Today, interacting with the new science of sports, is the software of teaching methods. These are limited by the enduring reality that genuine technique training still, often, collides with folk wisdoms. The central narratives of this book concentrate on non-traumatic training. But never forget the legacy of the old-ugly — the hanging on of drills battering boys and young men, hither and yon, in a very loosely justified simulation of some of the trauma of game action.

To an extent, the role of the contact-free conditioning drill excesses highlighted here, the sprints to no end other than "more," goes beyond any scientific logic found in medically certified kinesiology studies. Largely, this is because they are filling a vacuum left by former, palpably horrific, practices presumed to be dying out.

The granddaddy of them all is the *bull in the ring* drill. In this exercise, one player is placed in the middle of a circle of others who take turns hitting him. George Visger, a marginal NFL defensive lineman, including on the San Francisco 49ers just before they won their first Super Bowl, remembered the bull in the ring from his first year of Pop Warner youth league play in Stockton, California, at age 11. In that drill, he was knocked unconscious for the first of many times. Visger believes it was the start of the head trauma that would lead to nine brain surgeries, starting in his early 20s, for installations of and adjustments to a shunt to drain the fluids of his hydrocephalus, or "water on the brain." (Visger was one of the 21 named plaintiffs of the NFL's nearly billion dollars of payouts, continuing on a rolling basis, to NFL veterans and their survivors for various categories of brain and neurological impairments and death.)

Bud Wilkinson was a coach who won three national championships at the University of Oklahoma from 1947 to 1963. Regarded as one of the more cerebral members of his profession, he went on to run unsuccessfully for the U.S. Senate and to work as a television commentator. Wilkinson nonetheless is also credited with invention of the *Oklahoma* drill. In some places, this is called the *pit* drill or the *big cat*. In this case the pit is a narrow passageway in which a running back lines up behind an offensive lineman, who squares off against a defensive lineman for a kind of sumo wrestling free-for-all, in which they vie not to be the one who gets knocked out of the enclosed space.

Also still surviving in some places from the days of leather helmets is *man in the middle*. Here, a group gathers in a circle and a rotation of players gets called out individually for being on the receiving end of brutal shots. Of course, it's difficult to argue that all of these aren't reasonable facsimiles of game action. Or that practice doesn't make perfect.

In the *triple butt* drill, a runner and a tackler are set ten yards apart by a set of pylons that they are expected to circle around as they advance on each other. So, yes, there can be found brutality with a soupçon of mobility. Anyway, the tackler's job is to bury his head into the chest and midsection of the runner. They do this several times. Got to keep doing it until they're sure they have it right.

These drills and others go by different handles and with variations by locale. They also coexist with more sophisticated, technique-based drills that also are unavoidably, though at least not so gleefully, violent. In our supposedly more enlightened times, the drills usually are no longer quite as deceptively deadpan in addressing the finer points. There is a geometry to effective blocking and tackling, for maximum leverage and impact, and there is subtle education on how to play within the confines of rules strictures regarding use of hands and other factors. Examples of names of the better-rationalized drills include the *butt and press* and the *angle tackle*.

Then there are hybrids of contact with other players; of mere contact with the ground instead of with others; and of drills aimed at shedding inhibition and fear. In *monkey rolls*, players dive over pile-ups of teammates, one side then the other.

From time to time the intersection of old and new standards surfaces at a reckoning point. When this happens, ubiquitous social media usually plays an important part. In 2021, a minor uproar emerged over video that soon went viral of a snippet of a football practice session from two years earlier at the public high school in El Cerrito, California. The clip on YouTube showed what's often called the *machine-gun* drill. In it, a player is knocked flat repeatedly by a succession of teammates plowing into him, two at a time. In the grip of an embarrassing national controversy, El Cerrito High, in the notoriously "woke" San Francisco Bay Area, put the head coach, Jacob Rincon, on administrative leave. With the overwhelming support of team families and the community, Rincon was quickly back on the sideline, presumably minus the machine-gun drill.

One key to rehabilitation in such kerfuffles — what the larger society might now call avoiding "cancellation," football-style — is at least as much a matter of nomenclature as of content. For example, football practices have had an age-old drill for receivers often called the "noose" (or, in wordier form, the "settle and noose"). There's nothing violent or in any way objectionable about the noose drill itself. In it, pass catchers are merely practicing how to tuck away a completion as efficiently as possible in order to be able to turn upfield with the ball as quickly as possible. A 2009 YouTube video, narrated by the then head coach at the University of Nevada, Las Vegas, Mike Sanford, explained that the receiver is taught to position both hands circularly on the outside of the incoming ball before "noosing" or snatching it — "just like a noose would noose the neck of somebody hanging from it."

Again, the noose drill cannot get called out for being dangerous or otherwise bad in what it teaches. The only issue is that it has an obscure title, and not even an especially accurate or illuminating one. But the title does, arguably, echo the obscenity of the era of racial lynching in the southern United States, during which, of course, Black men were hung from nooses. And since the stronghold of football is the American South, two plus two equals five.

An army of lexicographers would need to be enlisted to research whether the title *noose drill* was indeed drawn from our lynching legacy, or in some less than conscious way was influenced by it. In another world, the noose drill might be called the snatching drill or the pinching drill (which sounds dumb, but really no more so than "noose"). Or maybe it's the case of there being no accident whenever something benignly athletic in football is portrayed with gratuitous aggression. "Is there something inherent in football making even the most innocuous skill aspects get identified in gross terms? Discuss."

As it happened in 2016, news reporters at the *San Francisco Chronicle* covering the background of Ted Agu's death alighted on an internal reference to the Cal team's use of something called the noose drill. Had they been consulted, the more football-knowledgeable writers of the newspaper's sports section surely could have informed their colleagues that this was a nothingburger. But in the organization of the news budget of a beleaguered contemporary newspaper, the sports people were being benched for this real-world story. The upshot was that the *Chronicle*'s newshawks' unspectacular find of a lurid thing called the noose drill set off a brief spasm of social media outrage.

Meanwhile, as they say in football, the *Chronicle*'s coverage, like that of others, was "leaving the ball on the ground"— fumbling the fundamentals — of Cal's cover-up of Agu's sickle cell trait and the team doctor's deception of the coroner.

Dangerous contact drills might be giving way to dangerous non-contact ones by degree. This thought arises every time a program gets called out for going overboard, either in a known abuse or in the report of it.

In 2022, Nebraska head coach Scott Frost bragged that his new offensive line coach, Dominic Raiola, had his charges vomiting "15 to 20" times each practice. "It's not because they're out of shape — he's just working them hard," Frost explained, with approval. "I think they love it. He's kind of freed them up to go be aggressive and I love the way they're coming off the ball."

When his remarks were not well received, Frost walked them back. Similarly, Cal conditioning coach Damon Harrington had embraced the mantra of punishment as a positive trait in internal communications, but he publicly disavowed the idea on the witness stand, in the face of legal liability. In his own second swing, Frost said he was just kidding. Player health and safety was a Cornhuskers priority: "Our training staff and weight staff are keeping me abreast of everything going on in practice." Yuk yuk yuk.

In a sport predicated on a narrow, but also undeniably functional, definition of toughness, football drills will always be somewhat performative in nature. At its feeder levels, hooking into boys' formulation of their identities, football's appeal to a cinematically unambiguous notion of manhood is uniquely well positioned to hook the impressionable and to abuse the vulnerable. As the 1930s Tin Pan Alley song said, *Ya gotta be a football hero / to get along with the beautiful girls.* The truth is that football is not for everyone. Peer pressure suggesting otherwise causes damage.

The monster on the field who is actually a teddy bear off it — the Sensitive Assassin — is one of the oldest plays in the hornbook of macho. Footballers provide more than their share of this archetype. In recent times, some athletes have gone a step beyond that, to a plea for a redefinition of manliness itself. Ronnie Lott, the San Francisco 49ers' Hall of Fame secondary guy, who was second to none when it came to "putting the wood" to an opposing player, in the vernacular, is one example. But many of Lott's post-career flourishes of gentility are aimed not so much at redefining manhood as they are at targeting safer-sporters in the grandstands. In his ideal world, he has said at public speaking appearances, every high school in the ghetto from which he sprang would have superior athletic trainer and medical resources. The ultimate goal for this crowd of thinkers might be a medivac helicopter hovering over every game and every practice. In football world, one is allowed to fantasize to a vanishing point; there's no need to pencil in costs and priorities.

Joe Ehrmann is a leader of a pack of ex-players taking the conversation in a slightly different direction. Ehrmann played defensive tackle at Syracuse University and went on to ten years in the NFL, starting in 1973, and three more in the United States Football League of the mid-1980s. Coming to believe that football's celebrated life lessons might be a bit skewed, he has devoted his later life to preaching a model he calls "strategic masculinity."

In addition to being named to the all-century football team at Syracuse (where he also lettered in lacrosse, also the second sport of the university's greatest contribution to football, legendary running back Jim Brown), Ehrmann is more proud of having been named a Most Distinguished Alumnus of the school for contributions to society. The Institute of International Sport put him on the list of the country's most influential sports educators. His area of special interest is preventing rape and encouraging the involvement of fathers in their children's lives.

Even, one would hope, in counseling sons that there are better ways to find empowerment and team-building skills than in wheezing and banging through gridiron glory in the American empire's last gestures of histrionics.

CHAPTER 6

Bringing
the
Heat

Mothers of soldiers the world over who get that knock on the door with the most horrible news, unimaginable news, are familiar with the process. For the mom of Braeden Bradforth, a 19-year-old offensive tackle, realization came in stages. No one from Garden City Community College called. There were only cryptic patches of reports from other loved ones who struggled to form the words. Even when they finally found a way to tell her that her Braeden had fallen, for good, in the remote southwest corner of Kansas, more than halfway across the continent, on the far edge of the next time zone, Joanne Atkins-Ingram couldn't quite process it.

In southern New Jersey, it was already well past midnight, early Thursday morning, August 2, 2018. A state employee on the brink of retirement, Joanne had just finished her volunteer shift at a homeless shelter in Freehold, where she helped out regularly. This was her first night back there in a while, since recovering from surgery. And the last days had been such a whirlwind! It was barely a week since Braeden — not yet sure just what he was supposed to be doing with his life after graduating from Neptune High School on the Jersey Shore — first learned that Garden City Community

College, of the Kansas Jayhawk Community College Conference, was invit-
ing him to play football for them. So it came to pass that a mere four days
later, Joanne was driving Braeden up the Garden State Parkway to Newark
Liberty International Airport, and seeing him off on a 6 a.m. American
Airlines flight to Garden City by way of Dallas. This was Braeden's second
time on an airplane. He hit the campus in mid-afternoon, submitted his
paperwork to various offices before the end of the deadline day, and moved
into the college's West Residence Hall.

In phone calls, Braeden told his mother he was settling into his dorm
and making friends. He bonded and played video games with C.J. Anthony,
a wide receiver from Atlanta. Anthony even somewhat resembled his new
buddy, all the way down to the dreadlocks.

On Wednesday, Joanne talked with Braeden twice, once in late morning and again in early evening. Braeden reminded her to send off the care
package she'd promised him — and not to skimp on one of his favorites,
Golden Oreo cookies. In the second call he said he was about to head off
to the second practice of the football team's first day. He expressed a little
concern that he might not be in the best of shape for what lay ahead. The
day before, Braeden had said some of the same things in a conversation
with his high school coach, Tarig Holman.

Before hanging up, Braeden said, "I love you."

"I love you, too, Tubby," Joanne said, using the family's nickname for
him. "We're so proud of you."

Near 1 a.m., after Joanne closed down her work at the homeless shelter
and was about to make the half-hour drive back from Freehold to Neptune
City, Braeden's older brother, Bryce, called. Haltingly, he said it was about
Tubby. He said police were at their house. Otherwise, Bryce was incoherent,
making no sense, and it sounded like he was in tears. Joanne was confused;
it didn't register, not consciously anyway, that Bryce was trying to communicate that something terrible had happened. She told Bryce that if he had
something to say, he should come right out and say it. But Bryce couldn't.

Joanne called her husband, Robert "Bo" Ingram Jr., Braeden and Bryce's
stepfather, a truck driver who was completing a delivery in Philadelphia.

She asked Bo what was going on. After an awkward silence, Bo said he'd find out and call her back. He did so a few minutes later.

"I don't even know how to say this," Bo said to Joanne. "Tubby is . . . gone."

"Gone *where*?" Joanne replied. Braeden had just arrived in Kansas. A gentle giant of considerable charm, with a unique relationship to his surroundings, he was notorious for his navigational eccentricity. But, after all, how lost could someone get on his third night on a junior college campus?

Then it hit her. By *gone*, Bo didn't mean Braeden was missing or lost. *Gone* meant *dead*. Somehow, in the stewardship of his new football coaches, the child Joanne had whisked off to Kansas for the adventure of his life hadn't survived 72 hours. She didn't yet know exactly what had happened, and as the evidence unfolded, it would become clear that she probably never would. But in that instant it finally dawned on her that Bryce's earlier shambolic demeanor was for the most tragic reason: his brother — her second son — had just perished, suddenly.

That's when Joanne Atkins-Ingram screamed, and everything went black.

At six-foot-four and ranging up to 315 pounds, Braeden Bradforth called to mind Michael Oher, the hulking Tennessean who won a Super Bowl ring playing on the offensive line of the Baltimore Ravens; Oher's extraordinary rise from foster care and homelessness was featured in the book and movie *The Blind Side*. Unlike Oher, though, Braeden had enjoyed a stable two-parent home life. He wasn't a good student, but he was a good soul. He loved children and was a soothing presence for not only his own dog, Duke, a pit bull, but also even the most snappy of his friends' pets. His bedroom on the second floor of the house in Neptune City was filled with stuffed animals. His dreads, flowing across the temples of his eyeglasses, and his goatee contributed to an aura of a bohemian, maybe some kind of frumpy intellectual, in addition to a happy-go-lucky jock.

Braeden's girth made him a natural to try football. And once he learned how to harness his size to a semblance of blocking technique, and not to hold back from hitting hard, he found he excelled at it. With her busy work schedule, and with Bo often unavailable on trucking assignments, Joanne managed to get her Tubby around to all his American Youth Football League practices and games by leaning on her network of local Facebook friends. Borrowing a page from Hillary Clinton, Joanne called them her "village."

At Neptune High, the coach under whom Braeden played, Tariq Holman, owned a quirky footnote in football history: as a cornerback for the University of Iowa in a 1998 game, Holman on successive possessions intercepted passes thrown by the University of Michigan's quarterback, the soon-to-be-legendary Tom Brady. In Braeden's senior year, Coach Holman helped him put together a highlight reel of his top plays. In addition to sending off hard copies of this video to recruiters for perceived possible landing spots, Braeden posted it on hudl.com, a website where football hopefuls seek to catch the attention of college athletic scholarship gatekeepers.

Unfortunately, Braeden got no bites. He thought his football journey might be ending with the All-Shore Gridiron Classic, a regional all-star game staged on July 12 at the high school field in neighboring Brick Township. From there, perhaps he'd enroll at an area junior college, and either play football or not. There was a regional junior college consortium team called the New Jersey Warriors.

In the spring of 2018, an assistant football coach from Garden City, Steve Shimko, had passed through South Jersey. At a track and field team practice, Shimko caught sight of Braeden throwing shot put and discus, and was impressed by his form, athleticism, and power. Over the summer, Shimko left Kansas to take a job as the assistant quarterbacks coach of the NFL's Seattle Seahawks. But he must have left a favorable report with his old colleagues, since on Thursday, July 26, Braeden got an email response from another assistant coach in Garden City. Would Braeden like to matriculate and play football there?

When Braeden shared the news with Joanne, he was over the moon. In the email from the assistant coach, Garden City wasn't offering a scholarship — but then again, junior colleges had open enrollment and only nominal tuition and fees.

One of the first orders of business for son and mother was locating Garden City, Kansas, on a map. For lifelong east coasters, this town with a population of less than 30,000 took the middle of nowhere to new levels. Garden City was located nearly 400 miles west of Kansas City, Missouri, more than 200 north of Amarillo, Texas, more than 400 northeast of Santa Fe, New Mexico. According to the Internet, Garden City had a good zoo and a claim to literary infamy: it and nearby Holcomb were settings of Truman Capote's classic nonfiction murder novel *In Cold Blood*. There were well-paying jobs in the meat-packing industry in Garden City, and it was becoming a place of surprising racial diversity. The school had a heavily enrolled English as a Second Language program.

After a Garden City admissions representative talked with one of Braeden's high school teachers, he and Joanne were off and running in a flurry of paperwork, preparation, and packing. They called the Neptune High registrar's office, and a transcript was dispatched. Braeden's local doctor, Kristen Atienza, gave him a rush physical exam and certified on the Preparticipation Physical Evaluation form that he was "cleared without restrictions." Dr. Atienza did add a note that his body mass index, 36.5, marked him as clinically obese and called for diet and exercise measures.

Late Sunday night, Joanne and Braeden made the obligatory shop at Walmart for last-minute items. Through the excitement of those days, Joanne also shared this family development with her Facebook "village." Friends weighed in both with tips and, materially, with fundraising for Braeden's plane ticket. Joanne acknowledged maternal tremors over sending her son from her nest so abruptly. She wondered if she was making the right decision.

"Don't worry, Joanne," one villager messaged back. "He's in good hands."

That last remark might not have been made if this circle of New Jerseyans knew that Garden City Community College was in the most turbulent period of its century-long history. Braeden Bradforth's football-focused landing spot was an institution out of control in every way.

Like many junior colleges, GCCC was an underappreciated local jewel, full of dedicated teachers on modest salaries who considered their jobs a calling, and bustling with bootstrapping young adults from underserved populations — not all of whom harbored profound academic ambition, but almost all of whom regarded their school as a gateway to better opportunities. But GCCC was going through a chaotic patch under its current president, Herman Swender. In 2017, the Higher Education Commission, the Chicago-based accreditation overseer, put the school on probation in the wake of a series of irregularities, all of them flowing from Swender's toxic leadership. His antics included toting an open-carry gun, threatening faculty and staff for speaking with journalists, searching their emails and cell phones, requiring prayers at the start of meetings, and in general administering a workplace rife with division and dysfunction. Three months before Braeden arrived on campus, the trustees commissioned an outside investigation of the Swender regime. Six days after Braeden died, the president's resignation would become official.

The school's athletic department, specifically, reeled with scandal. The director of the cheerleading squad, Brice Knapp, resigned amidst allegations of sexual harassment and abuse. One of the athletic directors passing through the revolving door, John Green, was found to have moved a female volleyball player into his house. There were outstanding complaints relating to Title IX, the federal law barring sex discrimination in educational programs. There were various allegations that could have led to athletic conference sanctions. There was a possible U.S. Department of Education investigation of financial aid violations.

Jeff Sims was the head football coach and also held the title of assistant athletic director. Sims was a nomadic but continuously employed figure on the college sports system's lower rungs. In 2016, he'd led the GCCC Broncbusters to the national junior college championship. GCCC marked at least the 11th stop in his football coaching career, including two separate stints as an assistant at Indiana University.

Sims also was a leading voice in the public debate over the structure of Kansas junior college football. Starting in 2016, a documentary series on Netflix called *Last Chance U* explored life in the sport's bottom-feeder programs. Like much of reality television, the series was simultaneously exploitive and oddly informative. The main theme coming across was that football-obsessed young men throughout the country, from hardscrabble backgrounds, were going to extraordinary lengths to nurture dreams of participating in the glory and riches of football's elite levels.

Housing top amateurs from ages 18 to 22 or so, the NCAA has around 125 Division I football programs alone, wherein an astonishing percentage of the more than 5,000 student-athletes have the goal — much closer to a pipe dream for the supermajority of them — of being drafted into the NFL. Below these are the NCAA's lower divisions. And below *them* are junior colleges, or JUCOs, under the umbrella of the National Junior College Athletic Association (NJCAA), where student-athlete goals differ little from those of the talent in multimillion-dollar college football factories. The only real distinction is that JUCO teams are largely comprised of the rejects from the more prestigious programs; these include players who simply couldn't get admitted to a four-year university because of poor grades or other factors. Combating food insecurity and lack of affordable housing options, some deploy desperate lifestyle strategies.

Even so, the grapevine promotes just enough anecdotes of the careers of NFL stars who used the JUCO path to word-of-mouth Hail Mary sustenance and success. For example, Tyreek Hill was a standout wide receiver at GCCC who wrangled a transfer to Oklahoma State University, and from there got noticed by NFL scouts. The connection of quarterback Patrick Mahomes throwing passes to the speedy, shifty Hill was a large part of the Kansas City Chiefs' Super Bowl–winning formula in 2019–20.

For Braeden Bradforth, enrolling at Garden City Community College meant punching his own ticket at Last Chance U.

Founded in 1923, the Kansas Jayhawk Community College Conference (KJCCC) was a long-time hotbed of JUCO football, in all its often charming small-time passion and fanaticism. In the 50-plus years since 1962, the conference had taken a step to contain those forces and keep its brands localized, by implementing a rule that no school could carry more than 20 football players from out of state. A similar cap regulated the other so-called high-revenue sport of men's basketball (where roster sizes are much smaller). But in 2015 the caps got lifted. Additionally, football team rosters on the whole were expanded from 63 to 85.[*]

One program quick to exploit the lifting of the cap was Independence Community College in Montgomery County — east of Garden City but likewise near the state's southern border with Oklahoma. On *Last Chance U* in 2016, the Independence football coach, Jason Brown, said, "We've got to turn over rocks and find kids at all costs." The next year, Brown's squad carried 69 players from outside the state. Meanwhile, in basketball, only 121 of the 540 men's players throughout the conference were Kansans (five of them hailed from the African nation of Mozambique).

Brown's counterpart at GCCC, Sims, was a fellow outspoken opponent of the cap. Sims framed it as rooted in racial discrimination, limiting the opportunities of young African-American men everywhere to find a foothold for their football marketability in the small towns of the Sunflower State. Despite the vocal opposition of Brown, Sims, and others, the KJCCC reinstated a modified cap a year after Braeden Bradforth's death. Today, no more than 55 members of the 85-man football rosters can be from out of state. This still represents a lot of the equivalent of football migrant labor: disproportionately student-athletes of color seeding the gridiron populations of largely white, rural JUCOs.

The misgivings Braeden expressed to his high school coach and to his mother about his preparedness for the start of GCCC practice proved prescient. Over the summer, other members of the team had received a package of schedules and instructions from Coach Sims and his staff, laying out their expectations for early conditioning drills and other responsibilities; the document was entitled "Garden City Football, Opportunity USA, 2018." Braeden, of course, hadn't seen it. Also, he was being dropped right into intensive conditioning drills with no accounting for the transition from the Jersey Shore, at sea level, to the half-mile altitude of the Kansas

---

[*] On the issue of the KJCCC out-of-state cap, but also on several other key aspects of the Braeden Bradforth story, I'm indebted to the excellent in-depth coverage of Sam Zeff of KCUR radio in Kansas City, a Public Broadcasting System affiliate.

high plains. On Wednesday, August 1, the temperature was 84 degrees with high humidity.

Braeden Bradforth, in less than tip-top shape, was a disaster waiting to happen.

At least two players, Johnny Jean and Kahari Foy-Walton, would tell the media that the ten coaches, one trainer, and eight student helpers who were present on August 1 either explicitly or implicitly denied the squad access to basic hydration. Later, GCCC's investigation would dispute this, stating that 60 gallons of water were on site and the student helpers had individual bottles in their carriers to hand out to anyone requesting them. The more subtle conclusion is cultural: Coach Sims's words and gestures likely discouraged water breaks. This was all in the tradition of football's vague but seemingly ineradicable code of prioritizing "toughness," an indispensable component of which was never betraying "weakness."

One player, Kirby Grigsby, said that while water was there, he and his teammates had the perception they'd be punished for partaking it. "If you got water, you were considered done. [That meant] it was basically over and you had to do your conditioning all over again the next morning." Grigsby further explained that Sims and his assistant coaches "said that water during workouts does nothing for you. It's how you hydrate 'before' and 'after.'"

The evening drills involved 36 sets of 50-yard sprints, with breaks of no more than 30 seconds between each one. As they progressed, a student assistant, Donte Morris, noticed that Braeden was wheezing. A fellow lineman, Olajuwon Lewis, running alongside, observed his dry mouth and his lips turning white.

According to some of the players, Sims taunted Braeden as he labored to keep up. His new friend, C.J. Anthony, may have been the only athlete on the field who actually completed his sprints at the required times (six seconds per 50 yards for skill position players, eight seconds for the others). Anthony noticed that the coach, who'd lent Braeden a pair of shoes to use at practice, yelled that he wanted his shoes back. Others corroborated this and added that Sims cursed and screamed that Braeden was "soft." At one point, Braeden fell to his knees and grabbed his chest; Sims ordered him to get up and continue.

Anthony: "I remember the pain on his face. He couldn't breathe. The coaches were telling him he was just being dramatic, to stand up. . . . I could tell he was out of whack. By the tenth one or so he wanted to stop and the coaches started chewing him up. Coach Sims was saying all kinds of stuff you never say in front of other players: 'Your dad says you work hard, but you don't.' Stuff no one wants to hear. You could see the pain in his eyes, like he wanted to cry, but instead of doing that he just sucked it up and kept going."

Anthony said he, himself, felt like he was going to die, "and I was in the best shape of anyone there."

The drills ended around 9:15 p.m. Braeden was the last in line leaving Broncbuster Stadium. An assistant who coached the defensive safeties, Caleb Young, saw him sitting in the stands with his head in his hands, and prodded him to move along. The team trekked the short distance toward the Dennis Perryman Athletic Complex for their first indoor gathering. Sims called it the "Winners Meeting."

After a few yards, Braeden stumbled off in another direction, toward the dormitory complex on the western edge of campus. It's unclear whether he was making a conscious decision to veer off. There was a brief exchange of words with Young, the upshot of which could have been either that the coaches were dismissing Braeden from the team or that he was resigning himself. In an email to school administrators nearly a month later, Young said he asked Braeden if he was quitting, and instead of responding with words, "he shook his head in what looked to me disappointment and continued to walk away."

Given Braeden's physical exhaustion to the point of critical illness, any conversation between the teenager and the coach, using either words or body language, couldn't have been very sophisticated. Braeden's prospective status on the team aside, he was in acute distress, yet was being allowed by the coaching and training staff simply to wander off. Indeed, in the wake of the grueling session, the trainer TJ Horton and his student assistants weren't bothering to check the welfare of *anyone*. They were busy breaking down equipment and putting it back into storage.

While the group convened at the athletic complex, it's speculated that Braeden tried to enter the West Hall dorm by the wrong passage, a locked door at the end of a narrow alley where the heavy air was even more choked. All that's known for sure is that he must have sat down in that alley and rested his head against the brick side of the building.

Back at the Winners Meeting, Young told Ben Bradley, the offensive line coach, along with head coach Sims, that Braeden had quit the team. Addressing the players, Sims sneered over Braeden's aborted Broncbusters career. "This kid didn't even finish the running today," the coach said. "He was slacking. He didn't even have a pair of shoes to lift in, but I gave him a pair of shoes." Sims said he felt disrespected and was directing Bradley to tell Braeden to "give me my shoes back."

The meeting broke up around 9:45. Routinely, the players showered back at home. A group of them walked toward the residential complex. Several, probably about five of them, spotted Braeden in the alley. The exact number of teammates gathered around is hard to say, since this was the first practice day and not everyone knew everyone else. Braeden likely had been slumped or lying there between 20 and 30 minutes.

Kirby Grigsby was one of them. Braeden "was in bad shape," Grigsby remembered. "He was trying to breathe. He was making like a humming noise as he was trying to breathe and I could tell he was not able to breathe like he wanted to. His eyes were closed, his tongue was sticking out."

In clinical terms, Braeden was "obtunded" — he had a dulled level of alertness and consciousness.

Someone hurried back to the athletic center, returning with Caleb Young, the assistant coach. Grigsby and others poured water into Braeden's mouth. Someone on the team staff — Young or another assistant — hosed down his body, evidently using a hookup at the side of the building, language in the subsequent Emergency Medical Services report would suggest. Young was reassuring the kids that Braeden would be OK. In that email to administrators a few weeks later, Young described "visible distress at this time however still breathing and making a stressful moan."

Young didn't call 911. Instead, he called head coach Sims for guidance. Sims told him to call Horton, the trainer. At 9:53, Young hailed Horton at home. Horton got there at 9:59. He didn't have 911 summoned, either, until 10:02.

EMS Unit 97, with paramedics Christine Macias and James Good, arrived with a screech at 10:10. In their report, they said "the coaches made all players go back to rooms so any witness(es) . . . were not present at this time." Braeden "was moaning and was wet. There was also a lot of water on sidewalk around him."

According to the report, "Coaches were only able to provide minimal patient history. Coach states patient had asthma and used an inhaler. Coach also stated he had seasonal allergies." Though Braeden's medical history included passing reference to asthma, interviews for a later GCCC investigation of the incident had no references whatsoever to asthma or allergies.

The EMS crew found Braeden unresponsive when they rubbed his chest. They measured his blood glucose level. He choked and started vomiting; Young would describe the upchuck as resembling "dirty motor oil." When the vomiting stopped, Braeden was loaded onto a soft stretcher and into the back of the ambulance. At 10:24, the medics designated a "code red" emergency.

At 10:33, the unit pulled up to the emergency entrance of St. Catherine Hospital. On the Glasgow Coma Scale, Braeden was deemed a 4 (a patient is considered comatose at anything under 7). Soon, his heart stopped. At 11:06, he was pronounced dead. A hospital pastor called the family in New Jersey. That's how older brother Bryce got word.

By then, head coach Jeff Sims was at the hospital. His message to the news media was that an emergency room doctor had told him of a test performed on Braeden indicating "a blood-clotting disorder." Sims said a blood clot likely broke free, traveled to his heart, and caused a heart attack. There's absolutely nothing in the records, contemporaneous or retrospective, coming anywhere close to supporting such a hypothesis. The medical records indicate that Braeden was administered something called a D-dimer test, which looks for the presence of a protein fragment known as a fibrin degradation. The D-dimer test had zero weight in the assessment of the cause of death. Notably, the preliminary report of the coroner's office — an intake document as the first steps of the autopsy were contemplated — had no reference to a blood clot. And everything intuitive — all that was observed and done on the spot, including the immersion of Braeden in water, by amateurs and professionals alike observing his critical state — pointed only to unanimous speculation, with near-certainty, that the cause of Braeden's collapse was exertional heatstroke.

Still, Sims stuck to his guns throughout that key initial news cycle, most effectively in an interview with *Sports Illustrated* online. *SI*'s article and other short items on the wire services framed the narrative of yet another sudden death, of a football player of no distinction, in a remote place.

Or as Sims put it: "Something that could have happened, anytime or anywhere . . . an act of God . . . "

The Finney County medical examiner's autopsy report took nearly four months for finalization and public release. The one-sentence summary of the 11-page report by the forensic pathologist, Dr. Eva J. Vachal, said it all: "*Considering the facts surrounding the case, the cause of death is judged to be exertional heat stroke.*" In the commentary, Vachal went out of her way to debunk the theory of a blood clot by writing that there was "no evidence of pulmonary thromboembolism."

By the time the report got filed in state court, on November 29, Jeff Sims's football team was in Pittsburg, Kansas, preparing to play the national JUCO football championship game against East Mississippi. I caught up with Sims that day on email.

The coach wrote back to me, in substantial part: "While newspaper head-lines may lead some to believe that Braedens Death [*sic*] had a connection with football or practice, it did not. It was unfortunate timing but truly is there ever a time that we expect the passing of a young man. Braeden passed away the evening after practice and we have been assured it was something that was out of our control. We all miss Braeden, GOD has his timing."

The GCCC–East Mississippi championship game was broadcast nation-ally on a tiered CBS Sports cable network. The Broncbusters lost, 10–9. The broadcast included no mention of the Braeden Bradforth death in August or the breaking news surrounding it.

In response to my queries, a spokesperson for CBS Sports had disclaimed any responsibility for the content of the upcoming broadcast. CBS said it was merely the carrier of the game; the producer was an independent company called Kitay Productions, which didn't return my messages. On December 1, I heard back from the company's owner, Joel Kitay. He explained that the delay had been caused by "being so busy getting ready to get on the air."

As to Braeden Bradforth, Kitay said: "Our announcers were aware of this, and it was discussed in detail when we had a phone call with the head coach prior to the game. It was up to the announcers to bring it up on air if the topic came up naturally in the flow of the game, which it did not."

By the time of the JUCO championship game, Sims had already accepted a promotion in the college football world. He was on the move again. Two days later, he became the head coach at Missouri Southern State University in Joplin, with a three-year contract — his 12th career stop. GCCC didn't clarify whether Sims's departure was fallout from the Bradforth death. Nor did MSSU clarify whether, in interviewing Sims for the job, he was asked to account for Braeden's death, or if the incident was even communicated to or factored into the decision of those who approved the hire. The *Joplin Globe* later would confirm that MSSU, unsurprisingly, knew all about the GCCC fatality on the prospective new coach's watch.

Sims coached only one season in Joplin before being dismissed, as the Bradforth death litigation unfolded in Kansas and as politicians and media commentators amplified the demand for answers there. Under his tutelage, MSSU won only two games and lost nine, so there was that. Even though dismissing Sims had fiscal implications, the university refused even to say whether or not he was being sacked, in the legal jargon, "for cause." (Sims was fired in December 2020, two years after he was hired. But the 2020 MSSU football season got wiped out by the pandemic.)

In 2022, KCUR radio's Sam Zeff reported that the NCAA's Division II Committee on Infractions had issued a 25-page report delineating violations at the MSSU program, "where compliance was an afterthought, if not entirely dismissed and disregarded. . . . Apart from directly committing and not addressing known violations, the head coach created and maintained an adversarial environment between his program, athletics leadership, and compliance professionals." To cite one example, an MSSU booster was enlisted to pay the back tuition bill for one of Sims's former players at GCCC so that he could transfer to MSSU. The report led to sanctioning the Missouri university with a reduction in athletic scholarships, a $5,000 fine, and three years' probation.

In the wake of the Bradforth death, GCCC undertook what it called an internal review. A later and more expansive investigation would expose the "review" as a sham, even worse than the cursory initial investigation by Cal after Ted Agu's death. GCCC's was driven by such testimony as Caleb Young's email memorializing the events of the fatal conditioning session and its aftermath. The report was haphazardly assembled by the interim athletic director, Colin Lamb; the campus police chief, Rodney Dozier; and a student services official named Tammy Tabor. The reviewers conducted no interviews and flatly concluded that nothing untoward had happened in the actions of college personnel.

Braeden's mother, Joanne Atkins-Ingram, and her friend and lawyer, Jill Greene, had no success in eliciting details or background from the GCCC administration. They were given, for example, conflicting information about the existence of campus surveillance video, which might have shed light on Braeden's wandering back to West Hall and the last hour of his life. In mid-August 2018, while making arrangements to have Braeden's belongings shipped back, Joanne spoke with Christine Dillingham, the office manager of residential life, who told her that wide-angle video existed of the stricken Braeden. However, college lawyer Randall Grisell, in response to attorney Greene's "spoliation" notice warning not to destroy possible evidence, claimed there was "no relevant reason" to produce any videos that might exist. Ultimately, the women were given the explanation that there was no surviving video, since surveillance camera footage, maintained by the campus police, got routinely overwritten every two weeks, an economy of limited computer server capacity. Why the college believed that video providing details of a death on campus was an immediate candidate for erasure will forever remain a mystery.

In late January 2019, Atkins-Ingram and Greene paid out of their own pockets to fly to Garden City. They visited the spot where Braeden collapsed, talked with numerous teammates and local witnesses, and ignited media coverage. Some of the stories moving forward would land in the Gannett chain's Asbury Park, New Jersey, newspaper, the *Park Press*, but there were also critical news and opinion articles published and broadcast closer to the scene of the crime. In November, a scorching editorial writer for the *Kansas City Star* had written, "If coach Jeff Sims had any awareness, he would quit coaching today." In March, opining on Missouri Southern State University's hire of Sims, the *Joplin Globe* editorial page would call for a full accounting by both the local institution and GCCC.

Just before Joanne left for Kansas, her New Jersey state senator, Van Gopal, wrote to the Kansas attorney general, Derek Schmidt, demanding an independent investigation of the death "and the professional practices of the Garden City Community College Athletics Department. This matter needs the force, authority, and expertise that only the Kansas Attorney General's Office can provide." Schmidt refused, claiming he lacked such authority.

In March, U.S. congressman Chris Smith, of New Jersey's Fourth District, got involved with a public letter to Ryan Ruda, GCCC's new president, advocating an independent investigation. Smith called Ruda's response to his letter "legalistic," "rude," and "condescending." In support of the campaign for an investigation, the Republican Smith later would pull together a bipartisan coalition of all 12 of New Jersey's House of Representatives members. They included Frank Pallone, a Democrat who chaired the powerful House Energy and Commerce Committee.

On the Jersey Shore in April, more than 100 friends and neighbors packed Asbury Park's Friendship Baptist Church for a town hall meeting to support Joanne's campaign for answers. Congressman Smith told the gathering he'd be introducing legislation for the creation of a commission to investigate the deaths of college football players. Smith also announced that GCCC president Ruda had agreed to meet with Joanne later that month. But the negotiations for the meeting would collapse over GCCC's preconditions; specifically, the college did not agree to share with her its "internal review."

The next month, the college released a page-and-a-half summary of the review. This claimed that the 84-degree temperature at the August 1 practice was seven degrees below normal for that date; that water, Gatorade, and ice towels were in abundance; and that no one saw Braeden falter during the drills.

In response to an overture from Congressman Smith, Kansas governor Laura Kelly weighed in with a letter — not to him but to Joanne. Kelly said she'd heard that Braeden "was a promising young man" and noted that she was herself a mother, "and I can only imagine the anguish you must feel." The governor, however, stressed that she had no role in the administration of Kansas community colleges, which are governed by elected boards of trustees.

In late spring, the GCCC trustees authorized an investigation funded at $100,000. Randy J. Aliment, of the college's outside counsel, the Lewis Brisbois law firm, and Rod Walters, a sports medicine consultant, were selected as co-authors.

Preparing to litigate, Atkins-Ingram and Greene retained a Kansas co-counsel, Chris Dove. In the end, the prospect of a wrongful death lawsuit was hamstrung by the Kansas legal doctrine of "qualified immunity" for state public agencies, which capped recoveries at $500,000. Eventually the parties settled for that maximum amount.

GCCC's investigation of Braeden's death, by Aliment and Walters, was published in October 2019. The 48-page report highlighted "a striking lack of leadership" by *former* college president Swender, *former* athletic director John Green, *former* head football coach Jeff Sims, and head athletic trainer TJ Horton. The report proceeded to lay out how their failures manifested in no oversight of the preparation for and execution of the fatal conditioning test, and in significant delays in response after Braeden was stricken.

Exertional heatstroke (EHS) is the leading killer of kids during football conditioning. The most foolproof way to save the life of a victim?

Immerse him in an ice bath, immediately. This is 100 percent effective in preventing death.

Supposedly, consciousness-raising and good modeling start from the top, where bad things happen to millionaire celebrity athletes. On August 1, 2001, Korey Stringer, a 350-pound offensive tackle for the Minnesota Vikings, died during training camp in Mankato, Minnesota. On July 30, the first day of practice, he'd left early due to exhaustion. The next day, Stringer willed himself to participate in drills again, and during the morning session of two-a-days, vomited three times. Afterward, in the air conditioned locker room, he became weak and dizzy. He was rushed to the hospital, lapsed into unconsciousness, and died in the early morning hours. This happened to be exactly two days before the death, chronicled in the first chapter, of the asthmatic Rashidi Wheeler at Northwestern. It was also 17 years to the day before Braeden Bradforth succumbed to the heat in Garden City.

With funds from her ensuing lawsuit settlement with the Vikings, Stringer's widow, Kelci, spearheaded several EHS initiatives to honor her husband's legacy. These efforts culminated in 2010 with the establishment of the Korey Stringer Institute at the University of Connecticut, which is dedicated to preventing sudden death in sports, especially from EHS. Unfortunately, when I contacted multiple officials from the institute for this book, none came forth with any data on EHS incidents or deaths. In the last chapter, I'll have more to say on how football safety studies, undertaken by think tanks and academic entities with ties to the industry, fall miserably short in disseminating pointed and useful public health information, much less in advocating effectively from such data.

One thing that can be said about EHS — in contrast with exertional sickling — is that it's distributed with racial neutrality; the main variables are the intensity of the heat, the size of the athlete, and the extremities of philosophy and safety inattentiveness of the supervising coaches and training and medical staff. One highly publicized victim of recent years was neither Black nor large. In 2017, 16-year-old Zachary Martin-Polsenberg collapsed during sprints at a football practice at Riverdale High School in Fort Myers, Florida; he was taken off life support 11 days later. His mother,

Laurie Giordano, set up the Zach Martin Foundation in his memory. In 2020, the state legislature passed and Governor Ron DeSantis signed the Zachary Martin Act, which mandates defibrillators and immersion tubs at game and practice venues. According to a 2019 report by the Florida Office of Program Policy Analysis and Government Accountability, there were 18 EHS cases at high schools in the state the previous year — and this survey didn't even cover football summer practices.

The 2010s were an especially taxing decade for American youth football EHS fatalities; seven teenagers died from this cause in Louisiana alone from 2012 through 2019. Whether this is an accelerating trend, compounded by rising temperatures from the global climate crisis, or perhaps merely a function of better reporting, could come into focus once pandemic disruptions of sports programs are fully in the rearview mirror.

In 2018, media coverage of the EHS death of the University of Maryland's Jordan McNair lapped many times that of Braeden Bradforth's a mere 49 days later. This was understandable, since Maryland is an NCAA Division I school. Additionally, McNair's narrative combined EHS boilerplate with the "toxic culture" overtones at Ted Agu's Cal. And in a rare and seemingly anomalous turn of events, several figures actually paid for their shortcomings with their jobs.

On May 29, McNair, a 325-pound offensive tackle, collapsed during practice. At the hospital, his body temperature was recorded as 106 degrees, and he was airlifted to a trauma center, where he got an emergency liver transplant. McNair died on June 13.

To his credit, the president of the university, Wallace Loh, issued an extraordinary statement that the institution "accepts legal and moral responsibility in the death of football player Jordan McNair." Nearly two and a half years later, the university paid a $3.5 million settlement to the McNair family.

Meanwhile, the larger accountability engine churned, by fits and starts. An ESPN report targeted the environment created by the football strength and conditioning assistant, Rick Court, where players were belittled and humiliated. It all sounded a lot like Damon Harrington at Cal. As one witness put it to ESPN: "I have heard players and myself called 'pussies' ior being unable to complete workouts and the constant foul language has become accustomed to our culture. It has been incorporated into how we spoke to our teammates and coaches, but it isn't seen as a negative because we are so numb to it now."

In the familiar pattern, the Maryland regents commissioned a study of the football program (it was prepared by sports medicine consultant Rod Waters, who soon would co-author the same exercise at Garden City). When the report was issued in September, the university cut loose conditioning coach Court, but the head coach, D.J. Durkin, remained on the job. Local and national outrage didn't abate.

On October 30, 2018, President Loh announced his own upcoming retirement the next year. (For technical reasons, his departure wound up not taking effect until the middle of 2020.)

The very next day, Maryland fired Durkin. In 2020, he latched on as an assistant to Lane Kiffin at Mississippi. In 2022, Durkin moved to Texas A&M as the defensive coordinator under Jimbo Fisher. With the passage of more time, Durkin's complete rehabilitation, in the form of another head coaching post, is considered not out of the question.

Almost exactly three years after Braeden Bradforth — on August 4, 2021 — Kansas junior college football recorded another exertional heatstroke fatality. It was strikingly similar, almost identical. Tirrell Williams dropped dead at Fort Scott Community College, 80 miles south of Kansas City. Like Bradforth, Williams weighed more than 300 pounds. Like Bradforth, Williams was 19 and African-American. After his transfer from a local emergency clinic, he lay in a coma for two weeks at University of Kansas Hospital in Kansas City, before expiring from the official listed causes of oxygen deprivation, septic shock, and muscle tissue damage.[*]

The college had told Williams's mother in Louisiana, Natasha Washington, that his hospitalization was precautionary. "I was never told that he was

---

[*]   Muscle tissue breakdown suggests the possibility of rhabdomyolysis from exertional sickling, but I wasn't able to determine whether Williams was a sickle cell trait carrier or if he was ever screened.

non-responsive," she said. Only when a hospital nurse told Washington that her son's condition was dire did she dig deep to buy a plane ticket to be at his bedside.

KCUR's Zeff reported that the incident stemmed from the Fort Scott head coach, Carson Hunter, discovering a candy wrapper on the field and proceeding to punish the whole team with a previously unannounced set of back-and-forth sprints. Coaches call these "gassers." Hunter added "up-downs," in which the athletes were directed to drop to the ground on their stomachs and pop right back up.

Tanner Forrest, the trainer, told Zeff that Williams collapsed, falling face-forward to the dirt, on "gasser number eight or nine." Coach Hunter stopped the workout briefly as two assistant coaches knelt to check on him. The drill resumed while Williams lay unconscious on the field. When a teammate tried to reach down and offer Williams water from a bottle, an assistant coach grabbed the bottle and angrily flung it across the field. Throughout the drills, there was no hydration in the 83-degree heat. One player said Hunter called withholding water a form of "paying dues," saying, "Water is for the weak."

By the time Forrest got to Williams, "he seemed to be having a seizure," the trainer said.

On August 20, Fort Scott's Twitter account posted: "Our Greyhound family has suffered a devastating loss. We send all our prayers, love, and support to the family of Tirrell Williams."

The board of trustees met days later. The minutes show that in the portion of the meeting devoted to athletic department updates, they discussed the installation of artificial turf for the baseball field, the start of the volleyball season, and COVID pandemic protocols. At the end, there was a brief mention of the Williams death.

In the middle of the season, Fort Scott abruptly ended its 93-year-old football program. In 2006 the school had played in the junior college national championship game under the same head coach, Jeff Sims, who'd go on at Garden City to win one championship plus gain another championship game berth. But by November 2021, Fort Scott had fallen on hard times in the win-loss column. In a statement that month announcing the termination of the program, the college said: "We simply do not have the resources to maintain a football team that would be competitive in the Jayhawk Conference."

President Alysia Johnston articulated her position at the next month's trustees meeting. "We could find nothing that we did that contributed to the young man's very unfortunate and tragic death," she said. Johnston added that "I believe with all my heart" that Coach Hunter regarded player safety as a priority. Later, trustees chair John Bartelsmeyer would tell public radio's Zeff, "I'm satisfied with the president and the athletic director and the administration." As for the incident, "Specifically, I can't say there's anything that has been brought up to change, other than to make sure that all of our athletes are — I hate to say the word taken care of — but overseen."

The athletic director and vice president of student affairs, Tom Havron, predicted "a great future of coaching" for Hunter. "He's going to do great things."

Garden City planted a tree to honor Braeden Bradforth. Fort Scott did nothing in memory of Tirrell Williams.

Carson Hunter landed a position on the football staff at the University of West Florida in Pensacola. As this book was being published, he was listed as the assistant coach for outside linebackers, and coordinator for the administration of the movements of student-athletes from school to school — newly facilitated under what NCAA procedures now call the "transfer portal."

CHAPTER 7

Time
to
Criminalize?

After Braeden Bradforth died, his father contacted the Garden City Community College campus police. This was Braeden's biological father Sean Bradforth, not Bo Ingram, the man who would marry his mom and become his stepdad. Sean Bradforth wanted a criminal investigation of the death of his son.

He had a point.

In my reading, at least two provisions of the Kansas Statutes Annotated (KSA) seemed pertinent. The first, KSA 21-5403, might be regarded as a bit of a stretch (but only with the proviso that it falls on proponents of "three strikes" incarceration to explain why that principle has been applied to serial shoplifters). KS 21-5403 defines murder in the second degree, which is the killing of a human being either "intentionally" or "unintentionally but recklessly under circumstances manifesting extreme indifference to the value of human life." Though surely no one actually wanted Braeden to die when he collapsed following the conditioning drills, a case could be made — and it's a non-trivial one — that the direct custodians of his well-being that night, in the employ of a GCCC program supervising his activity, couldn't have cared less whether their newest itinerant footballer from New Jersey lived or died. Certainly, no one paid any mind when Braeden, in obvious distress, broke away from the group into the hot Kansas night. Later, when teammates discovered him lying semiconscious, they summoned a responsible authority, an assistant coach, whose first thought was to call not 911 but the head coach. The athletic trainer, once on the scene, took three more minutes before calling first responders. All in all, there seemed to be at least as much energy invested in ordering the other student-athletes back to their rooms (the better not to be around to offer testimony) than in addressing the life-and-death matter right before them.

Grotesquely, Braeden, whose life could have been saved at an earlier point with a simple immersion in ice, got hosed down like some kind of chain-gang inmate. Had Braeden been a dog that died of such premeditated neglect, the Society for the Prevention of Cruelty to Animals probably would have raised more of a stink than did the college's powers-that-be.

A second KSA code, 21-5405, "involuntary manslaughter," might be accurate at a level a bit less metaphorical and more granular. KSA 21-5405 is defined as killing "recklessly" or "in the commission of, or attempt to commit" another felony or misdemeanor "that is enacted for the protection of human life or safety."

Needless to add, no such investigation, on either front, emerged from Sean Bradforth's entreaties to law enforcement authorities. In the Ted Agu death, the University of California, Berkeley, campus police assembled a 141-page binder of supplemental reports and interviews. There, it would become bureaucratically convenient to expand the reach of Ted Agu's death investigation and to hype it as a police matter. Eventually, it even became a legally useful tactic to term the collection of documents part of an actual criminal investigation (albeit one leading to no targets or prosecution), so as to ward off Public Records Act scrutiny. The university assured a court that "every" campus death got probed by campus cops, as a matter of "policy."

At GCCC there was no interest in nor utility to claiming or fabricating such a policy. When Sean Bradforth called, the campus police chief,

Rodney Dozier, merely advised him to try Michael Utz, chief of the Garden City police. The same Dozier would go on to co-author the college's initial whitewash no-interview "internal review."

"Chief Dozier said there was no report on the death of my son, which I found unbelievable," Bradforth told me. "He explained that the campus force had a very small staff."

According to Bradforth, Utz went on to say that the city police department had no documentation of the Braeden death incident either. Bradforth said the chief told him he'd both contact the Kansas Bureau of Investigation (KBI) and seek additional information from Jill Greene, Joanne Atkins-Ingram's lawyer. When Utz never called Greene, she called him, but made no headway in getting him to do an official probe. Greene also tried Derek Schmidt, the state attorney general, who never replied.

If Utz lied about calling Greene, then he also might well have lied in promising to call the KBI. But if the KBI did process some form of information from a local police department and documented it, that in turn would have undermined the later contention of attorney general Schmidt, to New Jersey state senator Van Gopal, that Schmidt's office had no jurisdiction in an investigation of Braeden's death and its background. The attorney general oversees the administration of justice throughout the state, and a local inquiry would have undermined plausible deniability.

Of course, buck-passing among public safety agencies is a common feature in touchy or unpopular investigations. More important for our purposes is the basic question: *Should* football conditioning deaths of this nature be matters of criminal investigation, rather than just administrative hand-wringing of one sort or another?

Sports is entertainment. Some clues are offered in the legal landscape of Hollywood make-believe and its expensive, infrastructure-laden productions. In 1982, actor Vic Morrow and two Vietnamese-American child actors were killed in a gruesome helicopter accident late at night during filming of a scene of *Twilight Zone: The Movie*. No criminal charges were forthcoming, though Hollywood did institute some new safety standards in movie productions. In 2021, actor Alec Baldwin accidentally shot to death the cinematographer Halyna Hutchins on the set of a Western film that was to be titled *Rust*; Baldwin said he had no reason to suspect, when he was rehearsing a scene of firing the gun, that it might be loaded with live ammunition rather than blanks. Fifteen months later, both Baldwin and the production company's firearms consultant, or "armorer," Hannah Gutierrez-Reed, were charged with involuntary manslaughter.

As with any hot-potato controversy around the locus of malfeasance, which can creep up to the line of that harder-core thing we call a crime — and in certain interpretations cross that line — this question cannot be dismissed as youth football conditioning deaths continue to pile up and scrutiny of football harm accelerates. How the question gets answered will not be a moot court dissection of the language of the law. The language is there. The answer, instead, will go to norms and political physics, impacting prosecutorial discretion.

In the most egregious cases, my own vote on criminal prosecution would be "yes." For any prosecution, the toolkit in evaluating whether to bring a case includes such factors as deterrence of future similar acts and a sense that the criminal process can serve the commonweal, regardless of the trial outcome. Willy-nilly prosecution is unwise, but with the right balancing of interests and values, even non-convictions can send useful messages on behalf of community safety and values.

The time is nigh to take that principle to the next level in certain avoidable deaths of young amateur football players. At the University of California, Berkeley, of football strength and conditioning coach Damon Harrington, special circumstances encompassed both his conceivable criminal negligence on the day of Agu's death and the background of Harrington's equally egregious incitement, three months earlier, of J.D. Hinnant's criminal attack on Fabiano Hale, after Hale's workout absence triggered extra punishment drill sets and a suggestion by Harrington that teammates hold each other accountable "by any means necessary." Those elements swirled throughout a fact pattern more compelling than the philosophical criminalization of a random "tragic mistake."

At Garden City, Jeff Sims lied about key aspects of the scenario, such as his ridicule of Braeden Bradforth throughout the conditioning drill and his awareness of the player's acute physical distress. Afterward, Sims also betrayed pernicious intent when he spread the false notion that Braeden had expired from a blood clot rather than exertional heatstroke. In a death narrative saturated with reprehensible, even disgusting, data points, those aspects of the coach's behavior were serious tells. All told, there were multiple benchmarks of quasi-homicidal action or inaction, all the way through the dereliction of duty prior to the belated 911 call. Finally, Sims's here-today-gone-tomorrow football coaching odyssey (which appears to have reached overdue inglorious finality at Missouri Southern State) gives an already foul mix the further suggestion both of the institution's belated and diluted sense of wrongdoing, and of his own absence of remorse.

Whether there's a technically applicable law — or, as the saying goes, there "oughta" be one — is something that's supposed to keep busy our deliberative legislative bodies, state and federal. Focusing on the possibility of criminal statutes for these deaths would be a better use of legislators' resources and tools than their momentary, attention-grabbing, and ultimately vaporous blue-ribbon studies of such anodyne topics as exertional heatstroke awareness. Put an imperial coach behind bars for killing one of his royal subjects? *That* might concentrate the mind of football world.

Even when legislatures mandate solutions, as in the new Florida law requiring ice tubs at the ready, their measures have the effect of increasing the costs, and hence the budgets, of the associated extracurricular activities. In practice, it becomes a budgetary blank check in return for bad behavior — the handing over of additional Monopoly money for the abstraction of a concept of safety. A better way would be to take responsibility for a threshold of well-judged costs, by rational consensus and in balance with other public priorities.

In the best-known area of harm, traumatic brain injury, new helmet technology and things like provisions for neurospecialists on standby have given rise not so much to a well-thought-through safety regime in the context of an educational institution with a plethora of academic disciplines and programs, but merely the featherbedding of "Concussion Inc." The slush funds trickle downstream from the profitable professional model all the way to strapped public schools. In the same way, our mess with the non-contact realms of football unsafety brings us to the threshold of "UnConcussion Inc."

So far there's only one known case of a football coach's prosecution for the reckless homicide of one of his players. The coach was Jason Stinson, at Pleasure Ridge Park High School in Louisville, Kentucky, in 2008. The player was 15-year-old Max Gilpin, who died of heatstroke. According to the classic article on the case, by writer Thomas Lake in *Sports Illustrated*, Gilpin was American high school football player killed in action number 665, at minimum, since 1931.

Lake chronicled the story of a boy who had wanted to abandon football as an extracurricular activity back in middle school, but was pressured by his parents to stick with it. His obedience to the wishes of his elders was eased by a growth spurt that took him to six feet, two inches tall and 216 pounds. With one of his girlfriends, a cheerleader, Max talked about his profound and ongoing ambivalence toward playing football. He said he had no appetite or instinct for football's aggression and violence, but adult authority figures steered him in that direction. On the Pleasure Ridge Park High Panthers practice field that fateful day, he was one of 104 aspiring players.

Coach Stinson, once an offensive lineman who landed a tryout with the New York Giants before getting cut, constantly pushed Max to be tougher and meaner. Stinson and his assistants goaded Max to stick his head right in there more effectively, to use his helmet as a weapon. Like Garden City's Jeff Sims and many others, Stinson liked to think of himself as more than a football guru; he was a life coach, a molder of young men who might be too lazy ever to amount to anything as adults, but for the prodding of a no-nonsense coach at an impressionable age.

At 5:30 p.m. on August 20, 2008, in 94-degree heat, Stinson shouted out instructions to the squad for the start of a new set of scrimmage drills. He had to repeat himself several times, with only a handful of the kids responding in more than desultory fashion. They dragged their feet and took their sweet time getting lined up. They had been working since early in the morning. They were physically exhausted and mentally fried.

"ON THE LINE!" Lake reported Stinson bellowing. "IF WE'RE NOT GONNA PRACTICE, WE'RE GONNA RUN."

When the players still didn't step right up to his satisfaction, Stinson's response was a punishment set of 220-yard — eighth-of-a-mile — "gassers," undertaken in football gear. The players took turns on the gassers for the next more than half-hour. At the later criminal trial, Stinson's defense attorney acknowledged, indeed proudly advertised, that the coach said, "We're gonna run till somebody quits."

One of Max's teammates, either motivated to impress the coach or simply angry at his unenthusiastic peers, sprinted through his gassers until he was gasping desperately. He got taken to the hospital.

And then another player quit. Just stopped running and walked away from the team. Stinson had found his quitter. Weeding out the quitters was a good thing. Quitters took up space where they didn't belong.

And then Max Gilpin collapsed and died. Between the mini-battalion of top players and also-rans alike at this practice, and those watching from an adjoining soccer field, there were nearly 150 witnesses to the event and its prelude.

When Stinson got indicted and tried, the Jefferson County community by and large rose to his defense. A silent auction was organized to raise money for his legal team. Character witnesses for *Commonwealth of Kentucky v. David Jason Stinson* included the school principal, David Johnson. He'd played football at the University of Louisville.

The jury found Stinson not guilty. With the exception of changing "every coach" to "many coaches," it was hard to quibble with the clinching line of the closing argument of defense attorney Alex Dathorne: "Jason Stinson on August the 20th of 2008 did absolutely nothing different than every coach in this county, in this Commonwealth, in this country, was doing on that day."

The commonwealth's attorney, Dave Stengel, told writer Lake that he knew going in that the chance of winning a conviction was less than 10 percent. "Football coaches are right up there with the Father, Son, and Holy Ghost," Stengel said. The article concluded that the case might have been "a kind of public-service announcement intended to make coaches be more careful. Which it did. Some coaches reconsidered their use of negative motivation, and the state passed regulations that required more first-aid training and better education on heat illness."

There's new prosecutorial precedent in sports other than football. On August 13, 2019, Imani Bell, 16, died at an outdoor girls' basketball conditioning drill at the Elite Scholars Academy in Jonesboro, Georgia, an Atlanta suburb. The temperature was in the mid-to-high 90s Fahrenheit. She collapsed running up and down stadium stairs, a drill more commonly associated with football practice, and died after her heart was twice revived in the emergency room. The Georgia Bureau of Investigation ruled the twin causes of death to be hyperthermia — calamitously high body temperature — and rhabdomyolysis, the phenomenon of the bloodstream becoming poisoned by dead muscle tissue during extreme exertion.

In 2022, Imani Bell's family came to a $10 million civil lawsuit settlement with the Clayton County Board of Education. In addition, the school's gymnasium was named after Imani.

A year earlier, a county grand jury had indicted the basketball team coach, Larosa Walker-Asekere, and her assistant Dwight Palmer. Clarifying charges of second-degree murder and child cruelty, the grand jury said the coaches were being held accountable for what happened to Imani Bell "irrespective of malice." As this book was being published, the criminal case was pending.

Rhabdomyolysis was covered here earlier in connection with the risks of exertional sickling for carriers of sickle cell trait. Commonly, rhabdo is the consequence of ES. You don't have to be a sickle carrier, though, in order to be felled by rhabdo. And separate from ES, rhabdo often compounds with or happens alongside heatstroke.

Just as you don't have to have a sickling vulnerability in order to succumb to rhabdo, so too can you be afflicted with rhabdo in a non-heat situation, just from overexertion. This is one of the growing areas of identification of coach abuse in conditioning. Experts are identifying "rhabdo clusters" in abusive programs, and the cases are beginning to capture wider public attention. To date, more than two dozen cluster cases have been documented.

In January 2023, five basketball players at Concordia University Chicago, in River Forest, Illinois, were hospitalized following a murky New Year's Eve practice episode. The team had just returned from two road games in California, during which some of the players violated curfew. At the practice, head coach Steve Kollar ran extra-intense sets of circuit drills as punishment for the violations of team rules. The previous season, Kollar had been coach of the year in the NCAA Division III Northern Athletics Collegiate Conference.

What was learned about the hospitalized players' conditions indicated rhabdomyolysis. In a letter to team families, athletic director Pete Gnan wrote, "Amid the already stressful and exhausting week, Saturday's practice represented a particularly high-intensity, collegiate-level circuit training." Gnan said that there were allegations that the intensity and difficulty were "a direct consequence of the broken curfew," adding: "Our athletics program has zero tolerance for harassment or retaliatory actions of any kind, and reporting mechanisms are in place for students, coaches, and related staff."

The same month brought related controversy to the football program at Rockwall High School in Heath, Texas. In a letter to the community, principal Todd Bradford said football coach John Harrell was placed on administrative leave pending a third-party investigation of an incident that left multiple players hospitalized with such symptoms as inability to bend, extend, or lift arms, dark urine, and sharp pain. Harrell directed an extra-period after-school class that effectively functioned as the football team's offseason conditioning program. There, in a punishment drill, the student-athletes were forced to do 300 pushups.

An estimated 40 lawsuits have stemmed from college football conditioning excesses. The granddaddy of rhabdo clusters occurred at the University of Oregon. As with the Sonny Dykes hire of Damon Harrington at Cal, the culprit at Oregon was culture change under a new regime.

In December 2016, Oregon lured Willie Taggart from the University of South Florida as the new head coach of the Ducks. Taggart brought along Irele Oderinde as his strength and conditioning assistant. From January 10 to 12, Oderinde directed drills of military basic training intensity. What would become a special area of scrutiny was the sets of pushups, situps, and up-downs prior to weight work. These were labeled as "warm-ups" and were supposedly designed to be capped at six to eight minutes. But on the days in question — near the very beginning of offseason winter conditioning — they lasted up to an entire hour.

Offensive linemen Doug Brenner and Sam Poutasi and tight end Cam McCormick were among those stricken. They were hospitalized with rhabdomyolysis. Poutasi sued the university and settled for $300,000. Brenner also sued Oregon, and his case actually went to trial in Lane County Circuit Court in Eugene. The parties settled in 2022, right after closing arguments and as the case was about to go to jury deliberation. During their trial testimony, Coach Taggart and conditioning assistant Oderinde apologized; they acknowledged that the extended warm-ups had gone overboard but insisted that the excesses were unintentional and did not constitute punishment. Oderinde had been suspended by Oregon following publicity of the incident, and just before his trial testimony, he was fired from his second stint at South Florida. Taggart left Oregon after that single year; he was the head coach at Florida State for two years, and at the time of this book's publication he had finished three seasons helming the program at Florida Atlantic University.

Doug Brenner's settlement sum with the University of Oregon was not announced. His lawsuit had sought up to $25.5 million. A separate effort by Brenner to build an additional $100 million liability bridge to the NCAA failed in court.

CHAPTER 8

The Oklahoma Kids

While it was a University of Oklahoma coach, Bud Wilkinson, who is given dubious credit in history for inventing the brutal "Oklahoma drill," it is a pair from the Sooners football athletic training and medical staffs decades later who have done more than anyone else to bring contemporary awareness to non-traumatic yet often fatal harm from training, and to push for standards and practices to curtail it. They are Scott A. Anderson, the school's former head athletic trainer, and Dr. E. Randy Eichner, once a football team doctor. (The Sooners' lead team physician, Dr. Brock Schnebel, worked closely with Anderson and Eichner, defending breakthroughs that challenged the prevailing sports medicine and public perception biases, and helping spread the word about exertional sickling.)

Anderson and Eichner continue with their advocacy in retirement. Separately and sometimes together, they compile data; expose individual abuses, often in real time; and propound needed reforms to peck away at the sport's unacceptable and ongoing recurrences of mortality and mayhem.

Perhaps their greatest achievement came when their writings about exertional sickling deaths led to the creation of an NCAA task force on

ES in 2007. Three years later the NCAA began mandating that its football programs offer testing for sickle cell trait in athletes — rolling out the program for Division I in 2010, Division II in 2012, and Division III in 2014. The number of Black players who actually availed themselves of this resource, rather than opting out and signing waivers, was unknown. In 2022, the NCAA took the additional step of eliminating the opt-out and requiring all athletes to document their sickle cell status.

The Ted Agu case in Berkeley showed that simple confirmation of the trait is no guarantee that attendant safe practices will be either internalized by a trait-carrying athlete or implemented by team authorities. Even so, it's undeniable that, as a consequence of the new screening regime, the number of college football conditioning deaths from ES has gone dramatically down, to near-zero. Whether it's exactly zero depends on if we can reliably count Agu's as the most recent one. In 2016, Eric Goll, a 20-year-old freshman football player at Chadron State College in Nebraska, died after the first day of conditioning. The forensics process played out in the familiar way, with an enlarged heart immediately getting tagged as the cause. Medical records then showed that a year earlier Goll had tested positive for sickle cell trait during a physical clearing him to play football at Florida A&M University. In 2014, he had experienced exertional heat illness symptoms after football conditioning day one. An NCAA Division II school governed by the testing mandate, Chadron State claimed not to know this history.

Another ES death was Quandarius Wilburn, 18, at Virginia Union University in Richmond in 2022. Litigation is pending there.

From the early sample size, a 2020 University of Washington study, published in the journal *Sports Health*, did conclude that the NCAA's legislation "may save lives." Unfortunately, at the same time, ES deaths at lower levels of football, often ignorantly labeled as something else, might well hover at the same historical rates. The most recent of which we can be certain was 15-year-old Trenten Darton of Aleda High School in Texas in 2016, but there are likely multiple others.

Anderson retired in 2022. He's a member of both the Oklahoma Athletic Trainers' Hall of Fame and the National Athletic Trainers' Association

Hall of Fame. He also has served as president of another trade group, the College Athletic Trainers' Society.

Anderson put his observations and research together with the medical knowledge and curiosity of Eichner, an internist and hematologist who left Oklahoma in 2009. The Anderson-Eisner consciousness-raising partnership had begun in 1996 with a fresh understanding of what had caused the hospitalization of Sooners wide receiver and kick returner Jarrail Jackson following an early season practice. Jackson suffered severe cramping and back spasms in what at first was assumed to be a heat-related event. In the hospital, he was found to be a sickle cell trait carrier, but it was only during his six weeks of prescribed rest that Eisner put two and two together, determining that the problem had actually been the little-noticed phenomenon of exertional sickling. (Jackson went on to play in the NFL and is now the head coach at Texas College in Tyler.)

Off and running in broader-based research and investigation, Anderson and Eichner would turn to a study of the more than two dozen NCAA football player deaths this century of the non-traumatic variety. As many as a fourth of them were in the first two days of preseason conditioning. They figured out that ES, whether or not so acknowledged at the outset, was the culprit in eight cases. It seemed clear that over a period of a decade, if not longer, ES had been the No. 1 cause of college football deaths, period. In talking with 20 African-American players past and present, they were able to tie what had been considered more generalized cramping problems to the specific risks associated with sickle cell trait.

In a chapter they co-authored in a medical research anthology, Anderson and Eisner noted that there are four clinical concerns for trait-carrying athletes, one of which is grave. The less serious problems include concentrations of blood in the urine and obstruction of blood to the spleen when at altitude. The one concern rising to life-threatening status is ES, which, if unattended, can spike to a fatal case of "fulminant ischemic rhabdomyolysis." Smatterings of cases, both fatal and non-fatal, find their most substantial cluster in football. They are also evident from time to time in basketball, boxing, and track.

The authors pointed to an "alarming" spate of NCAA Division I football deaths from ES:

> In the decade from 2000 to 2010, no death occurred in the play
> of the game or in the practice of the game. However, 16 deaths
> occurred in conditioning for the game: 15 in sprinting or high-
> speed agility drills, and 1 in weight-lifting. Of the 16 deaths, 4 were
> caused by sudden cardiac arrest, 1 was secondary to asthma, and
> 1 was due to exertional heat stroke (EHS). Ten (63%) of the 16
> deaths were tied to complications of sickling. Thus, SCT, carried
> by an estimated 3% to 4% of all these players, accounts for 63% of
> the deaths, an excess of 16- to 21-fold. The high intensity of football
> conditioning seems to play a pivotal role in many of these deaths.

As for the timeline in a particular deadly episode, Anderson and Eichner found that, in the face of maximal exertion, those sticky sickle cell clusters in the blood become evident quickly; some football players have collapsed from ES after only two to five minutes of sustained sprinting. In the major cases, rhabdo has caused death in less than an hour from heart arrhythmia or renal failure. The speed of deterioration in these ES cases is a tell that they are not classic heat-illness episodes. Simply put, the harder and faster the drill, "the earlier and greater the sickling," the Oklahoma researchers said. They concluded that the heat "is no more a trigger for exertional sickling than is unaccustomed altitude, uncontrolled asthma, a heedless fervor on the part of the athletes, or a reckless intensity on the part of the coach . . . Exertional sickling collapse is an *intensity* syndrome."

From retirement in California, Eichner beats the drum for saner foot-ball conditioning protocols in, among other places, a regular column for *Current Sports Medicine Reports* called "Pearls & Pitfalls." In these commentaries, Eichner, an admirer of the late novelist Kurt Vonnegut, packages his serious scientific findings in a droll writing and conversational style. Often accompanying his observations of scurrilous practices by coaches, followed by corrupt responses by institutions, is that fatalistic Vonnegutism, "So it goes."

"We in sports medicine ought to do more to help end these tragedies," Eichner wrote in 2018. "Football 'conditioning' is out of control and killing our kids." Three years later, in the course of chronicling no fewer than nine player deaths in a single summer — eight from exertional heatstroke, one from exertional sickling — he decried the "warrior culture" of some coaches, noting that all nine victims were linemen and "were at the mercy of demanding coaches in brutal heat. All nine were teenagers." He also laments the newly noticed incidence of group hospitalizations of athletes, likely collective rhabdo, following ultra-intense sessions — around 25 such scenarios are documented at this point.

Eichner doesn't like to bring attention to himself. He has consulted for around 50 wrongful death lawsuits, most of them in football but also others involving military or law enforcement or firefighter trainees. It was his alertness to Agu's details and timeline that prompted the family lawyers in that case to put together pertinent discovery and deposition testimony; these, in turn, led to revision of the official autopsy findings, with their tardy acknowledgment of exertional sickling .

No matter how you slice and dice them, conditioning deaths are dizzying not only in their cyclical predictability and absolute numbers, but also in the tacit takeaway of an unimaginable and unaccounted realm of sub-lethal damage. In 2020, Anderson co-authored a two-part study in the *Orthopaedic Journal of Sports Medicine*, which reviewed non-traumatic football fatalities in high school and college programs, as collected by the National Registry of Catastrophic Sports Injuries.* "Since the 1960s," the article concluded, "the risk of nontraumatic fatalities has declined minimally compared with the reduction in the risk of traumatic fatalities." Moreover, the articles found, non-traumatic fatality rates are significantly higher than — the most conservative estimate is "nearly twice as high as" — the rates of traumatic fatalities. The reason is that, across time, bans on spear tackling and improvements in care of brain injuries have driven reductions in traumatic carnage — even as deaths during "coach-supervised

---

* This registry, the NRCSI, is one of several official compilers of football harm data that followers of conditioning deaths call inadequate and sport industry–biased. More in the Chapter 10 discussion with football historian Matt Chaney.

conditioning sessions," the primary cause of which was "exertion-related fatalities," remained unchecked. Non-traumatic cases, the authors wrote, are "erroneously defined as not being directly caused by sport participation," a sentiment driven by a false implication of "individual frailty for which neither sport practices nor practitioners are deemed responsible."

In at least 36 cases, "Punishment was identified as the intent."

CHAPTER 9

Damar Hamlin: "The Brain Bone Is Connected to the . . . Body Bone"

On the December 1, 2022, Amazon Prime Thursday night game, a global streaming audience saw Buffalo Bills safety Damar Hamlin endure the ignominy of getting ejected for a dirty hit. "Dirty" is a loaded word. It was an illegal hit, for sure, one deemed by pro football's current rules regime to be egregious enough for sanctions in two forms: loss of playing time along with, in a sport defined by territory, the standard team penalty of 15 yards or half the distance to the goal line.

What happened was that Jakobi Meyers, a New England Patriots wide receiver, was on the verge of snaring a touchdown pass in the end zone when Hamlin blasted him helmet-to-helmet. That's a no-no and for good reason — though in the speed of an NFL game, it's often hard to figure out just how realistic it is to expect a player always to execute the presumably safer tackling technique called "heads up." This, or something like this, happens more than once in every game. Sometimes it's punished. Often it isn't. Here, it was "personal foul, unnecessary roughness." Blow to the head against a defenseless yadda yadda yadda. And Hamlin was disqualified.

This fairly standard play, accompanied by a penalty rather than a no-call, turned out to be the little-noticed opening act of a two-act passion play. Thirty-two fateful days later, during the ESPN Monday night game on January 2, 2023, Damar Hamlin didn't repeat the same mistake on a hard tackle in the field of play. This time Hamlin used textbook technique, leading with his pads instead of his encased cranium. The result was that he almost paid with his life. Yes, the tackle on Tee Higgins of the Cincinnati Bengals was a clean one. But with Hamlin's head properly kept out of harm's way, he left his midsection wide open for the full force of the impact.

Hamlin popped right up. A second and a half later, he collapsed motionless to the turf of Cincinnati's Paycor Stadium.

On national prime time TV, a first responder drama ensued, equal parts frantic and solemn. The only on-field fatality in league history had occurred in 1971, when Chuck Hughes, a Detroit Lions wide receiver, suffered a fatal heart attack while jogging back to the huddle. On that occasion, after Hughes got carted off, the Lions and the Chicago Bears played on. This one was different in the emotion and desperation on both sidelines. The athletes who accept shocking physical contact as their version of a day at the office could see that, this time, something was going terribly wrong. Hamlin was bleeding from the mouth, and his heart had stopped, and as the trainers and doctors worked furiously to revive him, Bills and Bengals players alike dropped to their knees, obscuring in a prayerful circle the TV camera's view of Hamlin and the emergency crew tending to him. In a coma, Hamlin was taken by ambulance to University of Cincinnati Medical Center. There, his heart lapsed into near-fatal arrhythmia a second time.

The game was held up more than half an hour. At first the show was expected to go on, as it always does. But once Hamlin's shaken teammates and opponents, having by that time retreated to the locker rooms, made it clear to league authorities that they were in no condition to resume, the game was canceled. The NFL had to scramble the TV schedule and the home-field advantage contingencies for the upcoming playoffs.

At this writing, Hamlin's diagnosis remained officially open. What could be expected from the clinicians of football world was a battery of tests and evaluations by redundant numbers of the most prestigious specialists money can buy. I'll take a wild guess here and predict that some of the doctors would agree that Hamlin was felled by a phenomenon called *commotio cordis* — more shortly — while others would not. In the football as well as in the tobacco industry, the manufacture of doubt is a precious commodity. Whenever possible, it's important to arrive at the most equivocal conclusion, and not only for the purpose of ameliorating malpractice claims. Every aspect of the management of the Hamlin story is aimed at the larger audience, for which certain findings of harm need to be sprinkled with less certain ones, cleansing the conscience. Acts of God are prioritized. In processing carnage, such factors as prima facie observation, intuition, and even the most informed hypothesis become discarded third opinions.

Commotio cordis, the syndrome that a national TV audience all but definitely saw unfold in real time, is a version of seemingly random cardiac arrest. But it's not random. The trigger is trauma to the precordium, the part of the chest covering the heart. Though not common occurrences, such events are far from unheard of. Scott Anderson, the retired University of Oklahoma athletic trainer who has researched football deaths and their causes at all levels, has isolated media reports and medical records for 12 *commotio cordis* football deaths since 1960. The most recent known fatality was Michael T. Ellsessar, a 16-year-old high school player in Sutton, Massachusetts, in 2010.

Anecdotally, former football players don't need to study medical literature in order know what this is about. Many recount their own scary episodes where someone took a hard shot in the wrong part of the chest at the wrong time. What followed was more than the sting of a bruised sternum.

In 2002, the *Journal of the American Medical Association* published the classic article on this syndrome. The lead author, Dr. Barry Maron, is a prominent cardiologist. Maron also has maintained a registry of chronicled cases and deaths. Some of them are not associated with football or any sport (such as the case of a teacher who got elbowed the wrong way while breaking up a playground scuffle). But 84 percent of Maron's 128 recorded events were in "competitive or recreational sports." In 16 percent of them, the cardiac arrest was fatal.

All this could have been grist for a focused national conversation on various guises of football harm up and down the system. Instead, a news media echo chamber, attuned to the NFL's irresistible storytelling, assured that an adoring public, already primed to process the official story, would encounter no such conversation in association with the Hamlin catastrophe.

The whole thing played out in a handful of news cycles. Within days, Hamlin, off a ventilator, then out of intensive care, then out of the hospital, was the latest of football world's triumphs in flipping the script. Once it was clear that he would live and not die, the flickering trope of "down with football" got transposed into enduring feel-good "up with people." ·

A hundred or so hours or so after the chattering class resonated with hand-wringing commentary on the collusion of millions of fans in gladiatorial spectacles with mortal consequences, abstracted to the point of decadence, an audience of millions woke up to: *He's OK, thank goodness. And who do you like in the playoff wild card round?*

While we were springing back from this communal trampoline, "Concussion Inc." did its part. Concussion Inc.'s demimonde of critics, with an inside-the-industry perspective, support research and critique with two main components. The first is deferring to football's existential violence by scrupulously shaping observations and recommendations in accordance with the assumptions of their audience. The goal is to make the sport, if not safe, then at least somewhat less dangerous. Like doctors advising patients not to smoke, drink, and overeat, they well recognize the limits of their ability to ward off bad human behavior.

The second component of Concussion Inc. is its research and development department. Always on the horizon is commercial hardware and software promising a less-bad end. A favorite is the better mousetrap, in the form of the better helmet. Another is return-to-play protocols that are fancy ways to formalize asking an injured athlete how many fingers you were holding up as he stumbled out of his stupor. Implicit in both prongs is the idea that if we can professionalize the measurement of harm, then we don't have to talk about it as much, and in the process we can spectate less guiltily as the gladiators play on.

Lost is the structural debate over who can play, under whose purview, and whether the public subsidies of this system, hiding in plain sight, should remain.

After the Hamlin scare, Concussion Inc. came right out of the box alongside the (helpfully momentary) hand-wringers. The *New York Times* published an opinion essay by Chris Nowinski of the Concussion Legacy Foundation. Nowinski played football at Harvard University before mugging for the cameras and throwing his body around in the professional wrestling exhibitions of WWE, where stunts like getting slammed onto tables caused serious brain damage, ending his athletic career. With the help of coverage initiated by Alan Schwarz of the *Times*, Nowinski went on to spearhead the harvesting of the brains of dead athletes (principally NFL players, but also football players at lower levels and participants in other sports), and raising awareness of dangers and propounding possible fixes. To his credit, Nowinski also opined about the need to limit youth football, but he had to be very careful about that part — his foundation had accepted NFL money, and in fundraising's tacit quid pro quo, had even bestowed on the league one of its annual meritorious service awards.

Post-Hamlin, Nowinski didn't use his *Times* editorial real estate to throw a forward pass for the restriction of football by age or level of commerce. If commenting on the NFL's feeder system, and the country's educational system that supports it, was on the table at all, this was not the time and place. Nowinski's essay was headlined "Football Is Deadly, but Not for the Reasons You Think." The sport's baseline of collision is indeed terrifying and leads to damage, Nowinski argued, but most of football's health costs are measured in traumatic brain injury and chronic traumatic encephalopathy. The etiology of the Hamlin case was an outlier.

Other takes in the *Times* through the same period included "We're All Complicit in the NFL's Violent Spectacle," "Fans Grapple With Football's Violent Pull," and "Why Do We Tolerate Football?" The *Washington Post* served up "Damar Hamlin is fighting for his life, and sports don't feel the same," then "Workers in dangerous jobs sympathize with NFL's Hamlin," and finally, succinctly, "Even Damar Hamlin's collapse can't make us quit our football."

Through the crisis, the NFL made all the right calls, minute by minute, by respecting the humanity of the moment, by scrapping the regular season "game of the year" between the Bills and the Bengals, and by making the hard decision to fudge the subsequent playoff schedule with the minimal disruption to the concept of competitive integrity. (Transparent advance data for the benefit of their newly joined-at-the-hip partners in sports gambling always have to be respected.) Of course, it's much easier to calibrate these choices in a society sated only by baked flour and hippodrome. And easier still with a happy ending.

A mere six days after Hamlin twice came close to dying, but thankfully didn't, his dramatic progress suffused Highmark Stadium in Buffalo with inspiration. There the Bills won their emotional final regular season game. By the next weekend's opening round playoff game, Hamlin was visiting teammates at the practice facility. Tweeted the daughter of an assistant coach: "I saw Damar today & bawled my eyes out! What a miracle to see him walking."

Across the country every year, communities stage bake sales to support families nursing severely injured teenage players. After that, the families are on their own. What costs catastrophic football injuries entail, insurance companies absorb, at the expense of general premiums. Those costs not covered by after-deductibles insurance, at that moment and then across time, the player and his loved ones pay. Or if they can't pay, they simply do their best to bury their medical deficits through the remainder of their educations, careers, and family lives. On and off the field, America has millions of such "lifer" ballers who also survived, but without a net.

Like many other NFL players as they become established and gain celebrity, Hamlin set up his own charity. His pet project was called the Chasing M's Community Toy Drive, and it had a crowd-sourced GoFundMe website. On the night of January 2 and over the next seven days, small and large donations poured in, raising its take from a few thousand dollars to more than $9 million. Hamlin's sensitive and canny distribution of this largesse loomed as the last piece of his journey to becoming a beloved mascot of football's community-shaping clout.

Unquestionably, Hamlin had a future career as an NFL ambassador, a TV talking head, and, depending on his temperament and public speaking skills, a motivational speaker. Did the options before him also include resuming his playing career? Early in 2023, a football doctor with whom I consult said exactly this:

"He was a top-fit athlete in full action. I am not concerned about three days on a ventilator for a guy like that. His first hospital stay in Cincinnati was only seven days and his second, at home in Buffalo, was only two days. As best I know, there has 'never' been a recurrent of *commotio cordis* in someone who survived it. So if that was indeed the cause, he could play again and his risk for CC would be no greater than the first time."

The missing piece of well-rounded social criticism of football world takes us past individual diagnosis, recommendations, and projections of outcomes. Will this jolt another division of Concussion Inc. into developing and requisitioning improved protective padding for the precordium? Such a new cottage industry would be in keeping with the culture's inclination to take no prisoners — that is, when it comes to fighting the last war.

Let's hope no such new piece of equipment emerges. Players are already armored up the wazoo. The only thing that could be accomplished by Chest Pad 2.0 would be to reinforce their already false sense of being bulletproof. Though few sports fans realize this, boxing's transition from bare knuckles to gloves made the sport far more lethal. Padded gloves protect the hand inside them more than the head they hit, and the diminished fear of broken hands made punches harder, faster, and more confident, worsening the damage at the other end.

The Hamlin episode was just the latest verse for the band that played on, stopping only for the NFL Players Association's anomalous muscle flex for a pause in the action.

For our larger society, it was another missed opportunity to map out all of football harm, body and soul. The children's ditty goes, "The knee bone is connected to the . . . *thigh bone.*" The corollary is, "The head bone is connected to the . . . *body bone.*" The problem of football lethality is *football.* Why, in any sensible rendering of assets and deficits, are kids put in harm's way to play it?

CHAPTER 10

Sudden
Death
Overtime

Matt Chaney, historian of football harm

That ultimate American curmudgeon H.L. Mencken never did observe, but maybe should have, that no one ever went broke overestimating the capacity of journalists to combine football cheerleading with empty-calorie reporting on the sport's devastating downside. Matt Chaney is among the few who refuse to go there. He breaks down the football problem succinctly. "Some jurisdictions outlaw tanning beds until the age of 21," he says. "You can't smoke cigarettes in the United States until you're 21. You can't drive a car until you're 16. Yet you're allowed to strap on a football helmet and ram each other when you're 5."

Somewhat less than nationally renowned, Chaney is an independent journalist and author in Missouri who's read and respected by a circle of reformed football veterans, public health researchers, and activists and opinion-makers keen on cutting a communal obsession down to size. He's our leading chronicler of the largely underground history of football harm. One of the things that make his work special is that it's more than just a herculean assemblage of rescued anecdotes and buried data. It's also social history.

Chaney points out that football became an ingrained fall ritual in the 1880s through our colleges. Originally this meant elite universities, the Ivy League schools, where the gentleman-gladiator persona became a fast track to Wall Street and the ruling class. The tropes and mythology of gridiron glory spread until they came to fit, hand in glove, evolving mass media technologies: first Sunday newspaper rotogravure color photo sections, then radio, then television. College football, along with sports that have since fallen from the top tier, such as boxing and horse racing, carved out the biggest slices of the sports spectator pie well before the NFL found its network TV footing in the late 1950s. (And always chugging along has been baseball, sentimentalized as the national pastime but seldom quite as profound in its marketplace and cultural penetration as hyped.)

Chaney's writings expose multiple, essentially unbroken and unrealized, cycles to rein in football's carnage. In the most dramatic example from popular history, President Theodore Roosevelt made the foundational intervention to "save" the sport from itself when he convened a summit of experts in 1905. This dog-and-pony show, whose real agenda was preserving the game rather than leading an assessment of it, has been replicated in numerous subsequent "safer sport" initiatives. Further, Chaney amusingly documents that the great Rough Rider — who had not played football himself yet extolled its virtues for all card-carrying male members of the human species — took care to privately steer his own four sons in the direction of other pursuits, even as his rhetoric for public consumption prioritized the sport over other supposedly effeminizing influences.

TR is but one blip in a timeline, long and deep, of high-profile fatalities and broken bodies, followed by feckless fixes. Sometimes the problem manages to peek over the horizon of media coverage. More often it gets downplayed or outright censored, in cheerful collusion with see-no-evil news consumers.

With deep dives into obscure local newspaper archives, Chaney collected what are likely the most comprehensive lists anywhere of youth football deaths and catastrophic injuries. Don't forget the latter, which include lifelong medical deficits — unrecognized by those enmeshed in football mania and thus, by default, subsidized by everyone else's insurance premiums and the health care system's frayed safety net. Among them are broken necks and other spinal damage, brain bleeds, and ruptured internal organs. One time I casually mentioned to Matt that my late father witnessed a football death at his own high school in St. Louis, which became part of a contemporaneous flurry to ban a blocking maneuver known as the "flying wedge." Immediately, Matt unearthed the newspaper clipping about the demise of Tommy Bagwell, Soldan High School, 1932.

Matt Chaney played football himself and loved it. He even co-authored a recently published history of his program at Southeast Missouri State University in Cape Girardeau.

"I had no pretenses going in — I knew it was 'kill ball' and that's what I enjoyed about it. But I don't recommend it for anyone's kid," he says. "Football is a thrill to watch and a thrill to play. The thing is, we'd all be better off if we acknowledged that playing should be confined to a minority of a minority. In any sensible construction of policy, not for juveniles."

While restricting participation would slow professionalized talent development, Chaney believes it also would relieve pressure on the adult levels, in the sense of at least being up front about the dangers. He counts among these hazards not only the familiar injuries and the more than anomalous death, but also another football world fact of life: abuse of painkillers and performance-enhancing drugs. That was the subject of his 2009 book *Spiral of Denial*, delving into the origin stories of steroids in football, possibly going back as far as some college ballers of the 1950s. Less disputably, Chaney proves the anabolic breakthroughs in the inaugural early 1960s seasons of the San Diego (now Los Angeles) Chargers in the old American Football League, under coaching innovator Sid Gilman.

Chaney calls football "our national drug." Quoting James Michener, he says the citizenry, by action and inaction, manifests an ongoing fanaticism that finds a way to pander to blinkered non-solutions. Consistently, we show a willingness to pay the price — or worse, to remain deliberately ignorant of it. Since no one likes to confront the sticker shock of the real full cost to our society, we keep two sets of books.

Chaney reserves special contempt for faith in safer, "heads up" tackling technique. For starters, as the 2022 Damar Hamlin episode showed, what gets protected in one part of the anatomy is part of a zero-sum game: some other part of the anatomy becomes exposed in the process. Viewed this way, football is chaotic life and death, and desperate measures to take it in another direction are just exercises in whack-a-mole. Most fundamentally, you have the factor that in real time — that is, real action on a real field of play, not in a theoretical safety construct — these blueprints for improvement tend to produce not safer football players but rather a cartoonish phantasm, an image of headless horsemen meandering sideline to sideline in a video game. To the extent that there's compliance with new mandates, the results are neither safe nor pretty. Players find themselves turning their facemasks to the side to avoid penalties. Meanwhile, "clothesline" tackles and other neck-high contact proliferate.

No one actually does it the way they're "supposed to" on a consistent basis. Because you can't in what Chaney calls "a forward-colliding sport."

Lies and damned lies

For purposes of my own reporting, I found the Chaney oeuvre invaluable for quantifying, but even more so for qualifying. In the moral equation, a bad outcome once is a fluke. Twice is a pattern. Thrice brings us to a threshold once of numerosity. Dozens in unabated iterations, where the bottom line is mortality or disfigurement? Now that's a societal sickness.

Somewhere between our medulla oblongatas and our cerebellums, we all know the shape of the problem. And at a certain point, the cult of precision plays into the hands of the apologists and purveyors of doubt. Infamously, NFL commissioner Roger Goodell once huffed that, after all, you can crack your head open slipping on a pool deck too. Long-time NFL and WWE doctor Joseph Maroon, one of the architects of the University of Pittsburgh Medical Center's profiteering ImPACT Concussion Management System — developed with the assistance of National Institutes of Health research grants — has tried to make the case that we should focus less on the kids endangered by football and more on balancing that danger against, say, the car accidents they might encounter driving to and from the football field. (In the movie *Concussion*, Maroon was the guy played by Arliss Howard.)

Chaney has used his own shoe leather to compile his lists, concluding that the recognized authoritative repositories of information, with industry bias, crab definitions of what was "football-related." In a decade-plus of scouring the same data banks somewhat less obsessively, I found myself nodding in agreement.

Much of this deficiency can be pegged to the National Center for Catastrophic Sport Injury Research, which operates out of the University of North Carolina. NCCSIR was directed for three decades by Frederick Mueller, an epidemiologist with graduate education degrees. The other face of the organization through some of the period before Mueller's 2013 retirement was Dr. Robert Cantu, the physician whose work with former pro wrestler Chris Nowinski and another researcher, Dr. Ann McKee of Boston University's CTE Center, vied with Dr. Bennet Omalu's for credit for catalyzing 21st-century conversations on the systematic braining of football players. NCCSIR describes its current structure as a consortium under Kristen L. Kucera, a Chapel Hill sports science and kinesiology specialist. The NCAA is one of NCCSIR's biggest funders.

The center finds that well over 90 percent of youth sports deaths and catastrophic injuries occur in football. That's the start of useful grist. According to Chaney, however, the total of such cases found in Google searches annually outpaces that in reports by the NCCSIR. Historically, Chaney argues, the Mueller group's methods had flaws infecting decades of statistics and conclusions. His last report, covering 2012, inaccurately proclaimed no "direct" fatalities in high school football, when available information definitively proved one in Tennessee and strongly suggested a second in Texas. Chaney says NCCSIR also missed cardiac arrest incidents and other "indirect" fatal illnesses. And there were 77 — not a mere 14 — survivors of catastrophic brain and spinal injuries sustained in football that year.

In 1974, two years before Chaney started playing high school ball in Hillsboro, Missouri, a boy named Brad Allen, who was obese, died minutes into the first summer conditioning session. At Southeast Missouri State in 1982, Chaney remembers injuring a teammate with a facemask hit to the midsection; "we both went to the hospital, and he was kept overnight, in agony." Two years after that, a friend and teammate, Chip Forte, died overnight of cardiac arrest following a scrimmage. Yet in 1985, when Chaney, still in college, began ordering microfiche sets of the Mueller accountings for UNC's NCCSIR, neither the Allen nor the Forte death was there.

As noted in Chapter 6, the Korey Stringer Institute was established in association with the University of Connecticut's department of kinesiology, nine years after the Minnesota Vikings player died of exertional heatstroke during conditioning in 2001. The NFL and Gatorade are partnership sponsors. When I asked the institute for statistics on juvenile football cases of EHS for this book, I was told it had none and I should contact NCCSIR.

The North Carolina center listed 47 high school EHS deaths between 1995 and 2017. Chaney counted 18 football deaths, traumatic and nontraumatic, in 2009 alone. Jumping ahead to 2015, another 13. All this before the brutal summer of '21 chronicled by Dr. Randy Eichner in *Current Sports Medicine Reports*. The NCCSIR's numbers fall short. Their data point choices shade the full truth, define deviancy down, and protect a multibillion-dollar industry Americans can't live without.

We need an autopsy autopsy

Fudging football's tragic toll is enabled by the nation's flawed autopsy system. Just ask the family of Ted Agu, who got a correct finding of exertional sickling only almost two years after the fact. Or the similar "a day late and a dollar shy" closure for the family of Aaron O'Neal at the University of Missouri in 2005.

"A teen football player dies suddenly in America, for reason unrelated to collision on the field," Chaney writes, "and the postmortem investigation produces more questions than answers — particularly whether the stressful sport contributed mortally." In 2009, Congress directed the

National Academy of Sciences to issue a blue-ribbon report on autopsy deficiencies, especially with respect to children. The resulting 300-page leviathan, *Strengthening Forensic Science in the United States: A Path Forward*, characterized the state of this public health space as "fragmented" and "hodgepodge," and promulgated multiple recommendations, mostly going to such aspects as ethical codes and standards of certification. Did the report make a difference? Has autopsy quality control changed for the better in the last decade and a half? The academy didn't respond to my multiple queries for an update.

Today's debate is novel — not new

Chaney's history is relevant to the current, bubbling-at-the-surface football safety dialogue. In his rendering, brain injury and overall juvenile safety concerns were front and center until the early 1960s, which happened to coincide with the start of the NFL's golden age. In 1907, the *Journal of the American Medical Association* opined, "Football is no game for boys to play." In 1951, consultants writing in the AMA publication *Today's Health* recommended the elimination of football below high school age. In 1954, the Educational Policies Commission of the National Education Association agreed.

But post the first entry of "greatest games ever played" — the overtime victory of Johnny Unitas and the Baltimore Colts over the New York Giants in the 1958 NFL championship game — the AMA walked back such negativity. In 1967, the group substituted touting "heads up" tackling for judging youth football. "As a kid, I only heard about the hazards of pot smoking. Brain damage from football? Nada," Chaney says. Only in this century did traumatic brain injury emerge again to become what NIH started labeling "the silent epidemic."

The 2014 Ted Agu conditioning death in Berkeley points to California's special contribution to the history of football harm denial. Fittingly, a key milestone came in 1905, the very year President Roosevelt was laboring to rescue the sport and its image.

In the 1870s, American football's antecedent, rugby school football, had taken root in San Francisco and Oakland. The teams were organized both by private athletic clubs and by area colleges and universities, spreading throughout the Bay Area. Churches and other institutions thrilled at the new collision football, which was more entertaining than soccer's mere "kicking," and games became staples of the social calendar. Newspapers supplemented their coverage of the contests with photos of female "beauties" in attendance.

In 1882, the *San Francisco Chronicle* — 132 years before it buried the lead of Cal's Agu death cover-up — commented sourly on the "healthfulness of the pastime." Four years later the sport served up its first local fatality: Berkeley law student M.E. Woodward, from a fractured spine.

In 1892, Walter Camp, the Yale player and coach who is credited as "the father of football," took his wares west, to Stanford. "The head or skull of a contestant is quite frequently called into service," the *San Francisco Call*'s M.J. Geary wrote critically. Camp rebutted: "Everything depends on the training. A well-trained and practiced football player rarely gets hurt. The danger to football players, properly trained and padded, is very small under the rules now governing intercollegiate games."

Which takes us to 1905, the year of Teddy Roosevelt. That November, Clarence Von Bokkelen of Santa Clara High School suffered a fatal brain bleed from a brutal hit during a game against San Jose High. Stanford president David Starr Jordan was even moved to order the dissolution of football at his university. Roosevelt-inspired rules tweaks came to the rescue.

Loving football to death

With the locus of football mania flowing downstream from the Ivy League, and with Jim Crow racial segregation having been dismantled in the South, no part of the challenge of depopulating football participation is more vexing than the love affair African-Americans have with this sport. And these are African-Americans at all levels of income and wealth. Today, the higher you move in the ranks, the more Black the game gets (on the field, that is — not so much in the head coaching ranks or front offices). A little more than an eighth of the country's residents are Black, but nearly half of all NCAA Division I players are Black. Sixty percent of NFL rosters are Black.

These choices aren't irrational, and the scolding tone of commentators on the so-called "Dr. J syndrome" skimps the context. (That term was coined in the 1980s to describe why so many African-American kids aspire to become National Basketball Association stars — including, obviously, those who had no hope of growing to the legendary Julius Erving's six-foot-seven height.)

"There is serious tracking happening with sports, by race and class," says David Karen, a sociologist of sports at Bryn Mawr College in Pennsylvania. "What do parents and kids perceive the sports opportunity structure to look like? People are going to gravitate toward opportunities that appear plentiful and well-used. Additionally, what kids choose to do in college is structured by what they'd had access to before — from very young ages onward."

At Hamilton College in upstate New York, sociologist Alex Manning studies the dynamics of racism, inequality, families, youth, sports, and culture. He says: "It comes down to how we treat sports institutionally. A lot of sports require substantial private resources in order to get to elite levels, but football is something supported and invested in by public schools. That's where the funneling happens."

Football's promoted benefits to the commonweal, such as forging teamwork and wider community-building, as well as time management and other disciplines said to be individual life skills, stem from the same structural determinism. Manning again: "Especially in the South — rural, urban, and suburban — football has become that rare open space and institution for Black youth-centered activity. It is where young African-American men can build recognition and attain some agency in their lives."

Passivity regarding the lethal risks of exertional sickling is an extra piece of the puzzle around football, racialization, and death. Oklahoma's Scott Anderson and Randy Eichner brought the issue to the forefront in recent years, but it's far from newly known. In 1974, after Polie Poitier died of ES while playing at the University of Colorado, a front-page headline in the *Kansas City Times* read, "Sickle Cell Anemia [*sic*]: Does It Threaten Black Athletes?"

Collectively, we couldn't all gloss over the complications of providing for both athletic opportunity and safety if the most conspicuous constituency didn't largely remain silent — even blissfully ignorant. This is just one more reason why the American juvenile football system, in the form of public high schools and colleges, has no business piggybacking as the NFL farm system. Lacking the national sports ministry often found in other countries, the U.S. lets the marketplace lay down the rules of the road; this leads to inflating claims of educational and community values in school sports teams, and downplaying public health values. By contrast, the franchises of European professional sports don't so co-dependently stock talent developed in schools.

Many Black people in or around football have expressed sentiments to me that could be summarized this way: "Why do we have to take the lead in raising sickle cell trait consciousness? That will just be one more thing used to stigmatize us and retard Black progress." Fortified by this non-messaging, some teen athletes, uninformed on the science, when compelled to screen, believe they're being targeted.

Activists for sickle cell anemia research and treatment don't help by not vigorously countering ignorance; they soft-pedal exertional sickling, fearing attention to it could draw oxygen away from their fundraising efforts for the full-blown anemia enemy. The Sickle Cell Disease Association of America (SCDAA) says, "Given the lack of scientific evidence that substantiates a significant correlation between sickle cell trait in athletes and training related sudden death, SCDAA does not support screening of athletes for sickle cell trait as a means to reduce heat related illness or death in athletes who are carriers." The parents of Ted Agu (who said they didn't know their own son was a carrier even though he'd opted into the NCAA-mandated screening and tested positive) might consider the link not insignificant. And greater awareness almost certainly would establish greater correlation.

The Centers for Disease Control (CDC) does recommend screening. It currently says: "Some people with SCT have been shown to be more likely than those without SCT to experience heat stroke and muscle breakdown when doing intense exercise, such as competitive sports or military training under unfavorable temperatures (very high or low) or conditions."

In 2016, when I acquired a stash of revealing deposition transcripts in the Agu death lawsuit against the University of California, I published them as an ebook. Wanting to give greater visibility to this information on Cal's cover-up, while at the same time avoiding the appearance that I was personally profiting from it, I got the idea of partnering with a sickle cell organization. I contacted SCDAA with a co-publishing pitch by which it would receive all royalties. The group's president at the time, Sonja L. Banks, responded enthusiastically and set up a telephone conference — then stood me up at the appointed time and disappeared. At some point in the interim, I speculate, she got the memo that sickle cell disease advocates were not supposed to be in the business of raising sickle cell trait awareness.

In 2022, the *New York Times* had an article about the reproductive calculations for partners carrying sickle cell trait. Understandably, the piece focused on sickle cell disease risks for trait-carrying parents, but there was not so much as a mention of exertional sickling. I queried the *Times* medical writer, Gina Kolata. She said, "I realize that people with sickle cell trait can have health risks [but] those risks arise under unusual circumstances. The vast majority with trait are unaware of it and have no medical reason to be concerned. The point of my story was that without testing people for trait, couples who are unaware that both parents have the trait can end up surprised by the birth of a child with sickle cell disease." What Kolata left on the table was the fact that a non-trivial minority of carriers *do* have medical reason to be more vigilant, given the phenomenon of careless, avoidable football player conditioning deaths at youth, non-professional levels, plus the disproportionate participation in the sport by African-American males. Economists would call "marginal" these differences between how knowledge of the trait could be utilized. Dismissal of the proportional importance of an aspect of the subject, while at the same time conceding that "the vast majority" were unaware of it, marked a lapse of journalistic mission. (More recently I tried asking Kolata if she thought the gene therapy breakthrough toward curing sickle cell anemia might relieve some of this tension and lead to a rise in the profile of exertional sickling. She didn't respond.)

Of course, this isn't all premeditated protection of the football industry. A restrained approach to sickle cell trait conflates with a measure of fatalism pertaining to all things football and public health. On the other hand, a similarly lackadaisical approach to tobacco would never have reduced the level of Americans who smoke from its high of 42 percent in 1964, when the surgeon general's report was issued, to today's 12.5 percent (according to the CDC).

Almost needless to add is that the remaining Americans who still smoke are also disproportionately African-American. All calculations of public health, it seems, were not created equal. In the Kansas community college football programs of the late Braeden Bradforth and his coach Jeff Sims, the hard-driving agenda of "Last Chance U" exists to maximize "opportunity." In that scheme, Blacks and football are partners in marriage — till death do them part. Exertional sickling denial is a microcosm of the public health trap football sets for all of us.

Toward a unified field theory of the problem of youth sports

The Greek ideal of a sound mind in a sound body is a cliche for a reason. Unfortunately, football obsession is a perversion, not a manifestation, of that concept. No responsible longitudinal study could demonstrate net positives from turning something so extreme into something aspirationally universal. In particular, the premium on bulk at the line of scrimmage, with specialists such as "run-stuffing defensive tackles," only makes the misappropriation of a theoretically good thing more stark; even leaving aside brain and other injuries, former football players in this category suffer disproportionately from heart disease and other health consequences of obesity.

Where it all starts is with the adults who run the asylum. Across the board, the American youth sports system has a way of turning children into adults and adults into children. In my reporting, I've observed the same unintended consequence in the enhanced opportunities for girls since the 1972 enactment of Title IX. For young females, especially in individual sports such as swimming, expansion of opportunity also inflated the space for sexual abuses by coaches. It's an ongoing dilemma of sexual politics and of the basic physics of human interaction in all walks of life. And it won't be easily eradicated.

Many critics believe the corrective is a labor-management model, in which the commercial values of sports get implemented more justly, by further empowering athletes at spuriously labeled sub-professional levels. I agree that this will distribute the spoils more equitably, but I disagree with its impact in the public health sphere. I once wrote a major magazine article on the drive to compensate college football players — bowing to the reality that they're not amateurs and that fictitious definitions to the contrary enable exploitation and inequality. However, I'm highly skeptical that new revenue opportunities for student-athletes, and new freedom of movement between schools, will improve the conditions of juvenile football. They're far likelier to incentivize the growth of the feeder system, to also incentivize juvenile football, when the national need is to scale it back.

For those parents who feel football is a good choice for their sons, no policy can (nor perhaps should) stop them. Enough good outcomes are out there to feed dreams, which seem to be our society's bottom line. The rest of us are content to enjoy the resulting entertainments, another bottom line.

Still, the evidence of football's dark side mounts. In a better world, stage parents could only take these pursuits to private clubs. In a better world, the blood sport of football would get off the public dole. Off our public fields. And out of our public schools.

The
Author

rvin Muchnick is author of *Wrestling Babylon: Piledriving Tales of Drugs, Sex, Death, and Scandal* (2007); *Chris & Nancy: The True Story of the Benoit Murder-Suicide and Pro Wrestling's Cocktail of Death* (2009; third and "ultimate historical edition" 2020); and *Concussion Inc.: The End of Football As We Know It* (2012). All were published by ECW Press. He has written many articles for the *New York Times Magazine*, Salon, *The Washington Monthly*, People, Spy, *Sports Illustrated*, and other major outlets, as well as for Ireland's Broadsheet and *Village Magazine* and San Francisco's Beyond Chron.

Muchnick's 2003 *Los Angeles Times Magazine* article, "Welcome to Plantation Football," helped spur the contemporary movement to compensate college athletes. His writings on deaths in the pro wrestling industry inspired a probe of World Wrestling Entertainment by the U.S. House of Representatives Committee on Oversight and Reform. His coverage of sexual abuse in global youth sports programs undergirded federal investigations of USA Swimming and of fugitive former Irish Olympic swimming coach George Gibney.

A former assistant director of the National Writers Union, Muchnick was named respondent of *Reed Elsevier v. Muchnick*, a landmark 2010 Supreme Court decision on the economic rights of freelance writers.

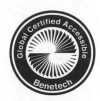

This book is also available as a Global Certified Accessible™ (GCA) ebook.
ECW Press's ebooks are screen reader friendly and are built to meet the needs of
those who are unable to read standard print due to blindness, low vision, dyslexia,
or a physical disability.

At ECW Press, we want you to enjoy our books in whatever format you like. If you've
bought a print copy just send an email to ebook@ecwpress.com and include:

- the book title
- the name of the store where you purchased it
- a screenshot or picture of your order/receipt number and your name
- your preference of file type: PDF (for desktop reading), ePub (for a phone/tablet,
  Kobo, or Nook), mobi (for Kindle)

A real person will respond to your email with your ebook attached. Please note this offer
is only for copies bought for personal use and does not apply to school or library copies.

Thank you for supporting an independently owned Canadian publisher with your purchase!